CW00729655

PENGUIN BOOKS

Feed
Your Children
Well

Joanne and Simon Blackley met while working together at Neal's Yard Bakery and Wholefood Restaurant in London's Covent Garden. Simon is co-author (with Rachel Haigh) of *The Neal's Yard Bakery Wholefood Cookbook* and now works as a freelance consultant and trainer, primarily with food-manufacturing businesses. Joanne was born and educated in the USA, where she took degrees in psychology. Since coming to England she has studied homoeopathy and completed her training as a psychotherapist. They have one son and live in North Yorkshire.

Feed
Your Children
Well

SIMON AND
JOANNE BLACKLEY

PENGUIN BOOKS

PENGUIN BOOKS

Published by the Penguin Group
27 Wrights Lane, London W8 5TZ, England
Viking Penguin Inc., 40 West 23rd Street, New York, New York 10010, USA
Penguin Books Australia Ltd, Ringwood, Victoria, Australia
Penguin Books Canada Ltd, 2801 John Street, Markham, Ontario, Canada L3R 1B4
Penguin Books (NZ) Ltd, 182–190 Wairau Road, Auckland 10, New Zealand

Penguin Books Ltd, Registered Offices: Harmondsworth, Middlesex, England

First published 1990
10 9 8 7 6 5 4 3 2 1

Filmset in 9½pt Linotron Melior

Made and printed in Great Britain by
Cox & Wyman Ltd, Reading

i

Contents

Introduction

We set out to write a book for parents who wanted to feed their young children healthily, not necessarily following any particular kind of diet, but preparing simple meals at home using fresh, whole ingredients rather than buying manufactured baby foods. We wanted to show that this could be done simply, and to explain *how* it could be done; what ingredients would be needed, what equipment, and how little time it really took. And for the benefit of those parents who were interested but unconvinced, we wanted to set out the arguments for this approach. To us, the nutritional, educational and social advantages of feeding a child with freshly made food seemed as important as the drawbacks and dangers of using manufactured foods.

Events have overtaken us. Starting with the Great Egg Scandal of December 1988, there has been a series of major food scares: following salmonella in eggs came listeria, possibly in soft cheeses and certainly in chilled foods, then aluminium in baby milk and bovine spongiform encephalitis in beef. Public concern about food issues is greater than it has been since the war. For the moment, at any rate, food is front-page news, and government ministers are setting up committees and 'reassuring the public' on a daily basis. Whether they will actually *do* anything which will materially improve the situation remains to be seen.

The furore over salmonella in eggs perfectly demonstrated the way in which attention can be diverted from the real issue. Mrs Currie courageously drew attention to a situation that is now, was then, and had for years been scandalous – 'most egg production' in the United Kingdom is infected with salmonella. In the days following her 'revelation' of facts which the Ministry of Agriculture had been aware of for many months, it became clear that some powerful people thought the real scandal was that a government minister should have 'unnecessarily alarmed the public', to the detriment of an industry which was 'an important national asset'. So persuasive did this point of view prove to be that the government hustled Mrs Currie out of office and quickly agreed to compensate the egg industry for the 'damage' she had done.

But the public *is* alarmed, and not unnecessarily. People want to know that they and their children are not being poisoned by the very food they eat, and are no longer convinced by repetitions of the bland assurance that 'there's really nothing to worry about'. People want action, and if the government cannot act quickly enough to satisfy them, then they will act themselves, by changing the way they eat. They will turn to fresh, unprocessed foods, and increasingly they will look for organically grown produce.

And now, as we complete the writing of this book, comes the appalling news that jars and tins of baby food and milk formula on supermarket shelves have been found to be contaminated by saboteurs with glass, razor blades and caustic soda.

Even before these recent scares, the expected arrival of a child would often stimulate parents to reconsider their own eating patterns, and rightly so. A mother's diet in the months of pregnancy conditions the development of the foetus and her own ability to breast-feed after the baby is born. Very soon the child will be eating the same food as her parents, and the quality of this food, and the eating patterns established in these early years, will profoundly affect her lifelong constitutional health. We wanted to help parents to think about and if necessary adjust their approach to the family's food – to the foods they choose to buy, to the way meals are prepared, and to how these are eaten and enjoyed.

Now it seems certain that large numbers of parents will be turning away in alarm from prepared baby foods, and will be starting to cook all their children's meals themselves. For those who simply want to know how to do this the recipes in this book, and the sections on Equipment and Food Ideas, will be useful. But we hope that the book as a whole will enable them to discover, through a return to a more traditional way of cooking which they may feel has been forced on them by events, the pleasure and satisfaction which come from regaining control over the preparation of one's own and one's family's food.

NOTE: We have chosen to refer in alternate chapters to a female child and a male child.

1 Food for the Whole Family

Attitudes to Food

Food and water, warmth and shelter: these are the three fundamental requirements for survival. The daily struggle to meet these needs absorbs the lives of several hundred million men, women and children. We in the 'developed' world are for the most part free of this sometimes desperate struggle for life. But if, in our comfortable sophistication, we allow ourselves to take our basic human needs for granted, we lose touch with a vital and enriching dimension of life itself.

In this age of the car, we tend to think of ourselves as cars. We make pit-stops to refuel with 'fast food'. We stoke up with the empty calories of refined sugar. We drink coffee for increased performance, and alcohol for lubrication. If we rest, it is in order to recharge our batteries. The market for special 'health' foods has flourished, as if perfect health could be achieved by tuning our intake of vitamin and mineral supplements.

But we are not machines; food is not fuel. The links between vitamin deficiencies and such disorders as scurvy and beri-beri have long been known, of course, and a total absence of any essential nutrient will certainly undermine health over time. But our bodies are organisms, not mechanisms. Their needs are of a complexity which defies mechanical comparison, and they are endowed with means of satisfying these needs which no machine can boast: a commonwealth of powerful and flexible self-regulating systems which can maintain the body's well-being under the most adverse conditions, drawing sustenance from a wide variety of diets.

Every individual is different, and no 'owner's manual', no set of dietary instructions can do more than provide the most general guidance. Indeed, to follow any rigid set of instructions may do more harm than good. Taste and appetite are the instinctive responses of our individual bodies with which we may react at a conscious level to regulate our diets. If I listen to it, my body will tell me what I should eat, when to eat it and when to stop. Its advice is not only free, but is also specifically tailored to my own individual needs.

Where food is plentiful and good, it is the breakdown of this relationship between head and stomach which is most likely to cause diet-related illness, and to learn again to listen to the voices of taste and appetite will provide the surest way back to health. Nothing in the general culture helps us. On the contrary, cultural messages tend to reflect and enforce our subjection to the neurotic impulses of self-indulgence and self-denial. This tendency is perfectly illustrated by the recent advertising slogan, 'naughty but nice', suggesting as it does that health and the enjoyment of food are actually opposed.

Healthy, satisfying and enjoyable food is essential to our psychological as well as our physical well-being. Food should provide not only nourishment, but in its role as one of the chief channels within a family for the expression of mutual care it should also provide recreation, relaxation and contentment. A newborn baby feels and knows his mother with his lips, mouth and belly before he knows her with his eyes. His primary relationship with the world is established through feeding. He finds that he has needs, and he learns that they can be met in full: the satisfaction of his hunger in his mother's arms assures him that he is not alone; that his fears can be soothed, and his discomfort eased. The satisfaction he derives from feeding will play an important part in establishing his lifelong capacity for contentment.

Family Meals

The shared enjoyment of food forges strong natural ties of loyalty and love within a family, as it does between mother and new-born baby. The members of a household are brought together from their different spheres and preoccupations for meals, and meet in the interval which mealtimes provide to refresh the ties of affection that hold them together by sharing with one another something which is both vital and pleasurable to each.

This does not mean, as we all surely know, that family meals are invariably sunny and harmonious occasions. The family table is a stage, and the play or ritual performed upon it can be a delightful playing-out of the care, love and respect felt by each family member for the others, or it can be an enactment of the control wielded or sought by one member of the family over the others, or of the battle for control between two or more members. As has already been hinted, control is a significant factor in our attitudes to food, and it is worth elaborating a little on this aspect of family meals.

Lack of psychological integration in relation to food appears to be endemic in our modern culture. Instead of responding to the inner compulsions of hunger and appetite, we tend to look outside ourselves for guidance in the choices we make about food. The widespread incidence of obesity, heart disease, intestinal disorders and other diet-related conditions is surely evidence of the breakdown of our ability to regulate our own diets in ways that promote our well-being. Disorders such as anorexia and bulimia are only the extreme manifestations in certain individuals of neuroses which we all share to a greater or lesser extent.

The characteristic feature of these neuroses is the dislocation of the automatic regulation of what and how much food is eaten. Lacking (or ignoring) the natural stimuli of appetite and repletion we seek to *control* our bodies as if they belonged to someone else; we indulge or we discipline ourselves. Loading a second helping on to our plate, we apologize for our 'sheer greed'; we say that we 'will probably regret it later'. Or we refuse the second helping, saying that we 'would love to but had really better not'.

It is not hard to see the ways in which this unnatural need to impose external controls on natural internal functions is likely to replicate itself among family members, and in the patterns and rituals of behaviour at shared family meals. Control can of course take many forms. Parents often divide between them the roles of denier and indulger; but it is important to be aware that constant pressure to 'go on and have some more' is just as controlling as constant grudging of every mouthful consumed. A father may seek proprietorial rights over the sharing of the spoils of his labour – and want the lion's share for himself. A mother may wish to control the division of the bacon which, if brought home by her husband, has only ever been cooked by her, and may want a favourite child to get the juiciest cuts (she will rarely seek them for herself). These are only examples, variations on a theme played out in every family.

There has, in the course of the last few generations, been a general breakdown of the formality of family mealtimes. We are probably all thankful that, except on special (usually public) occasions, and certainly in our own homes, mealtimes are now generally free from constricting rules of etiquette. But over this same period powerful external pressures on the family have arisen which have tended to replace the constraints of the Victorian parsonage with other, more modern, tensions.

The faster our cars and aeroplanes, and the more efficient and more numerous our time-saving devices, the less time we all feel that we have. One effect of the constant pressure of time has been that the daily preparation and enjoyment of food have been squeezed from their central position in the life of the household and have become less and less valued, both by the culture generally and by families themselves. (This does not apply to the prestigious *haute cuisine* of dinner parties or other special meals, nor to special 'health diets'. But it *does* apply to the regular daily routine of ordinary family cooking.) Family members, locked into timetables imposed by the demands of school, job or other commitments, are increasingly unable or unwilling to meet together even once a day for shared meals. Women, who still bear the major (and often the sole) responsibility for the purchase and preparation of food in most households, even when they also go out to work, are increasingly unable or unwilling to devote more time and energy than is absolutely necessary to an activity so poorly appreciated by society and so undervalued within the household itself.

At the same time, the food industry has developed and aggressively marketed a vast range of new products, supposedly in response to customer demand for foods which give greater convenience and greater freedom of choice. With pot-noodles, boil-in-the-bag *coq au vin*, frozen TV dinners, pre-cooked pizza and a host of other goodies stored in cupboard, fridge and freezer, and with the aid of such technical innovations as microwave ovens, each member of a household can eat different food, at different times, and in different rooms. Set mealtimes fragment, the distinction between meal and snack breaks down, and the occasions for eating multiply. This is the 'convenience' and 'freedom' which, apparently, we have chosen. The phenomenal rise in the consumption of meals outside the home, and in the purchase of prepared meals for consumption at home, has certainly been good for the food industry. But have these developments really been so good for the consumer? Nutritionally, the enormous increase in the consumption of fats and sugars in snacks and fast foods has been a disaster. Perhaps even more important, though, is the way in which these changes have alienated us from our food, and from one another.

The birth of a new child provides an opportunity for the members of a family to reconsider their food choices and their eating patterns. It should be taken as an opportunity to place an appropriately high value on the quality of the food brought into the home, on the care devoted to its choice and preparation, and on the social interactions involved in its shared enjoyment at family mealtimes. If buying and cooking fresh ingredients in preference to prepared meals, both for children and adults, requires a sacrifice of what is currently seen as convenience or freedom of choice, the nutritional and psychological rewards for the whole family will surely outweigh it. But our intention is to provide in this book recipes and methods that meet all the requirements for convenience of a modern family, and we believe that to choose each of the ingredients of a meal, and to determine and control the method of their preparation and combination, is to enjoy greatly *increased* freedom of choice in relation to food.

We stress the importance of involving children as early and as closely as possible in choosing foods for the home and in the various processes involved in preparing them for the table, as well as in the family meals themselves. But it is important that all the adult members of a household take part in this central aspect of child-rearing. The major responsibility for the family's food may fall on one parent, but it is essential that the other should take an active part, however small this may be, in *all* elements of the food cycle. A man who contrives to establish that any aspect of this work is simply 'not my job' avoids the challenges and deprives himself of the rewards of cooking for a family, and misses an opportunity to teach his children that to feed oneself is among life's greatest satisfactions. Similarly, it will be hard for a child to learn the vital lesson of the enjoyment of food when an important member of the family demonstrates his or her indifference or displeasure by continual absence from the regular family meals.

A child learns by example far more readily than he does by verbal explanation or command, and every effort made by parents to examine and balance their own attitudes to food in the years and months leading up to the birth of their child will be repaid many times over in terms of the ease with which they will be able to teach the child healthy eating patterns.

Appetite, Taste and Preference

Hunger and its satisfaction, rather than indigestion and its relief, constitute the rhythm of a healthily regulated diet. Appetite is the body's way of matching its consumption to its needs, and if we are never aware of hunger we will have no sense of appetite, and will allow our eating to be controlled by greed, by anxiety or guilt, or by social or marketing pressures.

A child's tastes and preferences should always be respected, but this is not to say that his whims should always be indulged. Disordered eating patterns in an adult (whether recognized as such or not) are often characterized by a sense of the opposed, and sometimes alternating, pulls of self-indulgence and self-denial. So with a child the natural balance of health, maintained by a continuing cycle of hunger and satisfaction, can break down at an early stage if the parents' aim is to regulate his intake of food to meet some preconceived notion of their own, rather than to respond to his appetite in ways that give him satisfaction.

Beware of setting up, either in your own minds or in the patterns of food-related behaviour established between you and your child, the idea or model of a stark choice between indulgence and denial, between being 'in control' and 'out of control'. From the earliest days of breast-feeding onwards, there is likely to be a strong impulse, whenever a difficulty arises, to deal with it as a straight choice between 'being tough' and 'giving in', and particularly so if this is the way in which you make your own food choices. What is necessary, on the other hand, is to respond appropriately to the needs of the individual child at the specific moment.

The problem may be to do with a night feed, a refusal to eat a meal you have prepared, a sudden demand for chocolate biscuits, or any one of a myriad of situations that arise in the course of the childhood-long negotiation of food issues between you and your child. There is never, in any of these situations, a right course or a wrong course of action. 'Being tough' cannot enforce a desired type of behaviour in the child, and 'giving in' cannot jeopardize it; and certainly neither one course nor the other will guarantee his health. It is an appropriate response that is required. To attend to the promptings of your child's appetite and tastes, and to respond appropriately to them, will not only be to give him what his body needs, but will also teach him to value his inner feelings and enable him to attend and respond to these promptings himself as he gets older.

What is an appropriate response? Again, there is no sure answer to this in any situation. What is certain, however, is that only by *attempting* to respond appropriately to your child, and by experiencing his satisfaction when you succeed, can you begin to learn how to relate to, and understand, his real needs. This requires openness at all times to the messages your child is giving you (not necessarily in words), and willingness to respect and consider his demands before ruling them out simply because you had something different in mind. You will only be able to respond to his needs appropriately if you are first aware of your own, are ready to accept that the two do not always coincide, and are prepared to judge impartially between them when they conflict.

We are not suggesting that in every instance you will be able, or should even try, to meet each need your child voices. Nor are we saying that your own needs as parents should never be considered. What we are saying is that, in relation at least to his food, your child's needs should never simply be ignored; that, for the sake of his present and future physical and psychological well-being, it is important that his tastes and his appetite are allowed to develop in an atmosphere of acceptance and respect.

Until a child is able to talk and to articulate his needs, and particularly in the first few months of life, it is often difficult to be sure exactly what those needs are. In order to make an appropriate response to a baby's inarticulate wail of distress you will have to distinguish, for instance, between a genuine need for food, a demand for affection, and an expression of discomfort. Do not expect breast or bottle, or a piece of bread, or any favourite food, to cure all ills, or use it as a substitute for some other thing that a child really wants.

The use of food or drink to pacify a bored, lonely or uncomfortable baby or child will teach him to eat for comfort. The confusion of food with unrelated elements of a child's life may also lead to the development of extreme food likes and dislikes, which are usually a response to a situation set up by his parents: an expression of rebellion against inappropriate parental coercion or control, or of a desire for the recognition of needs that have been ignored. Extreme likes and dislikes should always be treated with sympathy and respect. Forcing a child to eat something he does not want will always be found to be counter-productive. The situation must be examined coolly and carefully to try and work out what is actually going on: are you really sure that your child is simply 'being naughty'? Put yourself in his position; think back over the events of the day, or of the past week, and try to imagine what he might be trying to tell you through his behaviour.

Extreme food dislikes (and extreme likes are only dislikes in reverse – the refusal to eat anything *other* than the chosen food), when they persist and spread from one food to another, are a major disruption of the development of healthy eating patterns. You will not be able – and should not try – to force a way through such an obstruction. The only course is to back away from it, by removing any pressure which might increase the violence of the child's reaction, and then to build a path around it, by uncovering and relieving the underlying distress which led to the difficulty. This is unlikely to have any direct connection with the particular food itself.

What characterizes the extreme dislikes we have been talking about is their persistence, and especially their ramifications. Of course, a child may show a pretty violent antipathy to a particular food simply because he does not like its taste. It is worth remembering that although your child's tastes in food may differ from yours, it is unrealistic to expect him to eat anything which you find totally unpalatable. Similarly, he will almost certainly want to try any food he sees you eating with obvious pleasure.

Bargaining with Food

Another common error is to use the power of giving or with-holding food as a means of rewarding or punishing a child for its behaviour. Again, this confuses food with other elements of the child's life, and jeopardizes the development of the easy and natural relationship between his physical needs and his taste for foods that will satisfy them. Bargaining with food teaches him that his inner feelings, which as a baby constitute his entire sense of himself, are respected and cared for less than his ability to match his behaviour to external and alien standards, and that his need for food itself can give neither pleasure nor satisfaction, but is in fact a terrible weakness, putting him for ever under the power of others.

If this sounds like an overstatement of the case, it is perhaps only because the use of food as currency in a constant bargaining between parent and child is so widespread that we have become inured to it. It is surely both tragic and cruel, however, to cut a child off from the enjoyment of food *as food*, perhaps for the rest of his life, by teaching him that it is a prize which must be either earned or stolen.

The lines along which this tragedy is acted out are surely familiar to us all: 'Come on now, and when we get home you can have a nice drink'; 'Yes, of course you can have a chocolate biscuit, but not until you've tidied your room'; 'If you shut up,

I'll give you one'; 'I told you, no ice cream if you're naughty'; 'Eat this up first, and then you can have some pudding.' Using food to strike a bargain in relation to food itself (as in the last of these examples) doubly reinforces the message that food is concerned not with meeting internal needs but with meeting the expectations of others.

Try to recall your own childhood. Was the power to give or withhold food used as a means of persuading or coercing you? Perhaps you still reward yourself (for a hard day, or for cutting down on sugar) with food treats, or deny yourself food pleasures as a form of self-punishment. Perhaps you still feel guilty about (or simply find it difficult to enjoy) eating your evening meal unless you feel you have really earned it.

Our ability to choose the food we need, and to derive from it its full capacity to satisfy, nourish and sustain both the body and the person as a whole, depends upon our ability to take a straightforward pleasure in what we eat *as food*. A healthy enjoyment of food – and therefore a healthy diet – is threatened when values are placed upon it other than those associated with its flavour, texture, bulk, digestibility and (for adults) its known nutritional value, method of production, and perhaps country of origin. The natural development of a child's eating patterns will be thwarted by attempts to bribe him with the promise of food, or to punish him by withholding it.

Understanding Food

We have made the point that a healthy diet requires not only wholesome food, but also a wholesome attitude to food. A working understanding of food and food issues is essential both for the making of good choices and for the confident enjoyment of the full physical and psychological nourishment that food should deliver. Understanding requires both information and familiarity. We do now have better information than in the past about most processed foods (although this applies only to those we buy for home consumption). But the recent concessions made by the food industry, after long and intensive pressure for better nutritional labelling from groups representing consumers, leave one curiously dissatisfied. We now know the proportions of saturated and unsaturated fats present in most processed foods, but what are we to do with that information? It sometimes seems that the better informed we are, the more confused we feel.

We may now be in a position to choose between two brands of powdered soup on the basis of their relative fat content, but this does not enable us to choose between either of these manufactured products and a pot of home-made soup. There is no way of thinking about the packet soup and the home-made soup *as foods* which would enable us to compare like with like, and we can only make a choice between them on grounds of convenience. Indeed, the fact that one of the packet soups is low in saturated fats may persuade us (quite incorrectly) that it is actually 'healthier' than anything we could make for ourselves at home using fresh ingredients.

A large part of the problem is that the manufacture of many of the highly processed foods we eat nowadays bears no relation to anything we might do in our own kitchens to transform raw ingredients into finished food. The design and manufacture of a modern food product is incalculably technical. We may recall that butter is made simply by churning cream, but margarine is a hi-tech mystery. In this context, a list of ingredients – or even a full table of nutritional information – is something of a red herring; the product remains alien to us.

This alienation will be proportional to our lack of familiarity with the ingredients of our foods as whole, unprocessed agricultural products. When you regularly prepare family meals, starting with basic whole ingredients, you begin to wonder what 'modified starch' and 'hydrolysed vegetable protein' actually are, and why so many flavourings and flavour-enhancers are needed in processed foods.

What becomes clear is that the principal ingredients of most highly processed foods are not themselves fresh, whole, unprocessed foods at all. They are instead refined, and therefore stabilized *commodities*: easily traded, transported, stored and handled. Fresh, whole foods are live foods, and are therefore perishable. Unrefined flour, sugars and oils, all of which have clear nutritional advantages over their refined equivalents, are liable to deterioration. The large-scale manufacture and nation-wide distribution and sale of processed foods *require* the use of nutritionally inferior ingredients.

We are not going to suggest a return to some imagined pastoral idyll of self-sufficiency. The recommendations in this book are made in a full awareness of the pressures, constraints and complexity of busy modern lives, but they will involve the use of fresh raw ingredients in preference to processed and packaged pre-prepared food products. Geoffrey Cannon states forcefully the reasons why the food industry exerts its best endeavours to persuade us otherwise:

Food manufacturers do not want to poison the population: of course not. Corpses do not eat. The problem is that generally speaking, it is not whole, fresh food, but highly processed food with its 'added value', that makes the money. From the business point of view, a potato is small potatoes. Better, is a chip. Better still, is a crisp. Best of all, is a Crunchy Waffle.*

The answer of the food industry – the small group of massive companies that dominates the manufacture of highly processed foods – to criticisms such as these is always, 'Well, you know, we're only giving the public what they want. If people didn't buy our products we'd soon go out of business.' However, real food choices have to be made within the constraints of availability, time, income, social and marketing pressure, and under-standing. The point is that the food industry has a powerful influence over the conditions within which we as consumers make our food choices. Not only does it possess an awesome strength in the marketplace, spending around five hundred million pounds a year on advertising (and accounting for a quarter of all television advertising), but in the realm of govern-ment legislation on official food policy it constitutes a persua-sive lobby. Geoffrey Cannon researched in detail the connections between the food industry and UK government advisory committees on food and health, and concluded that between 50 and 60 per cent of the members of these committees were 'people who are (or were) employed by, funded by or advisers to the food industry'.

---

* *The Politics of Food*, Century (1988), p. 17.

We will shortly be looking more closely at some of the nutritional benefits of fresh foods and some of the dangers of processed foods. For the moment we will simply state our belief that, even leaving nutritional considerations aside, there are inherent advantages in choosing, wherever possible, fresh rather than processed foods. These advantages concern *attitudes* to food; they have to do with familiarity, understanding, confidence and self-empowerment in relation to food, and will play an important role in the food-related education of your child.

Food Additives

Food additives – colourings, flavourings, preservatives and other 'modifiers' – constitute only one form of food adulteration. Other forms include the addition (or artificial retention) of water to increase weight, or of air to increase volume; the presence of chemical residues from agricultural fertilizers, herbicides and pesticides; and contamination by micro-organisms.

We have seen that the use of refined, and therefore nutritionally inferior, ingredients serves the interests of the manufacturers of processed foods. Adulteration from contamination (whether by chemical residues or micro-organisms) is clearly not in the manufacturers' direct interests, but it *is* in their interests to avoid as far as possible the costs of preventing such contamination. The addition of extra air and water has been practised by the baking trade for centuries and has been brought to a state of near perfection by modern baking techniques. The obvious advantage (to the bakers) is that a factory-baked 800g white loaf not only looks bigger than a traditionally baked wholemeal loaf of the same weight, but also – since it holds far more water – contains proportionately less expensive (but nourishing) flour. The retention of water in meats and meat products by chemical means is another common modern practice. Adulteration by the addition of non-food chemicals – whether or not these can be proved to be harmful – is *always* done to suit the manufacturer and, however forcefully the industry may argue to the contrary, confers no benefits whatsoever on the customer. In all these cases the maximizing of profits takes priority over public health.

Of the 277 regulated additives used by the UK food industry (many of them restricted or banned altogether in other parts of the world), only 149 have the 'E' prefix to their identifying numbers, indicating European Community approval. Manufacturers are also free to identify additives by name rather than number (for instance 'amaranth' instead of E123 for the purple colouring used in jams, soft drinks, yoghurts and fruit pie fillings, which is associated with cancer and with hyperactivity in children*), and they often do so, having found that there is less customer resistance to names than to numbers. The health hazards, of course, remain the same. These range from asthma and migraine to epilepsy and cancer.

The dangers from the residues of agricultural pesticides arise from the consumption of small quantities of toxic chemicals over a long period; commonly used pesticides include many chemicals suspected of causing cancer, miscarriages, birth defects and allergic problems in this way.† The nitrates used in agricultural fertilizers, which also leave residues in some foods and find their way into drinking water (as well as being added as preservatives to many meat products), are similarly thought to be carcinogenic.‡

Although the direct link between a chemical and a disease is often impossible to prove (because the toxic effects are generally chronic rather than acute), a substantial body of scientific research has certainly established 'reasonable doubt' about the safety of permitting unrestricted quantities of these chemicals in human food. One would expect the bare possibility of such a widespread risk to public health to be enough to justify the introduction of legislation to restrict the use of some of these chemicals, but successive governments have been reluctant to put the health of the country's citizens ahead of the interests of its chemical, agricultural and food-manufacturing industries.

---

* London Food Commission, *Food Adulteration and How to Beat It* (1988), p. 55.
† ibid., pp. 86–94.
‡ ibid., pp. 112–15, 134–6.

This is not the place to enter into a detailed description of the possible hazards to health of each of the different permitted food additives, or of chemical residues, or of viral and bacterial contamination. The most accessible source of reliable, up-to-date information on this and other aspects of food is the London Food Commission, 88 Old Street, London EC1V 9AR. The LFC is an independent source of research, information, advice and education on food and public health, whose interests cover all food matters from production to consumption.

Baby Foods

The dangers of any form of food adulteration are much greater for children than for adults. The still-developing digestive and immune systems of young children make them far more vulnerable to any kind of toxin, and acute toxicity may result from exposure to dosages which would only be of cumulative danger to an adult. Particular problems of child health associated with chemical adulteration of foods include hyperactivity, asthma, eczema and allergic disorders.

There is no government legislation in the UK outlawing the use, in foods likely to be eaten by babies and young children, of colouring agents, many of which are known to be dangerous to the health of some adults. Instead, the food industry operates a voluntary ban on their use in 'special' baby foods. This applies only to foods intended for babies up to the age of twelve months, and does not of course include the many foods which, although not specially made for them, are nevertheless designed and advertised in such a way as to be attractive to children, and which therefore form a significant part of the diets of many children, and may even be given to some under the age of twelve months. On some brands of fish fingers, for example, the coating contains annatto – E160b – for which safety tests have not been completed, and which causes skin rashes in some people.*

The manufacturers of special baby foods are of course aware

---

* ibid., p. 57.

of the vulnerability of the children who eat their products. It is doubtful if the voluntary ban on the use of colourings in these foods would ever have come about without the growing public disquiet at their use, particularly in children's foods. But the manufacturers are naturally keen to capitalize on their 'phil-anthropy' in operating this voluntary ban, and the fact that their products are 'free from artificial colourings and preservatives' is usually displayed prominently on their labels.

There is no way of knowing whether these manufacturers also apply particularly stringent quality controls to the raw ingredients used in making their baby foods, to ensure 'safe' levels of agricultural chemical residues. Only one manufacturer that we know of produces 'organic' baby foods, which are indeed of a high quality but are around three times as expensive as their non-organic equivalents.

There have been at least two cases in recent years of the contamination of baby foods by micro-organisms. The first, much publicized at the time, involved the British manufacturer Farley (since taken over by Boots), which was forced to recall stocks of its dried milk powder after a number of cases of food poisoning among children were linked with the product and the source of contamination was located in its factory. This was followed by the more recent scare of early 1988 when Milupa, a leading manufacturer of powdered, ready-mix baby foods, similarly made public announcements on the radio, recalling certain of its products after the discovery of salmonella bacteria in one of its factories. In both cases, prompt action by the manufacturer did much to limit the damage done, demonstrat-ing the sensitivity of baby food manufacturers to the danger that their products could be responsible for food poisoning in young children.

Ironically, the risk of food poisoning caused by contami-nated processed food has probably increased with the reduction in the use of chemical preservatives in their manufacture. The food industry in general is coming to rely on modern packaging techniques such as vacuum-packaging, on freezing, and (if it has its way) on the supposedly 'safe' irradiation of food with nuclear isotopes, to replace the sugar, salt and chemicals it has traditionally used as preservatives, all of which have recently met sharply increased customer resistance on health grounds.

New preserving methods may in part account for the increase of more than 250 per cent in the annual number of reported cases of food poisoning in the UK over the last ten years.* It may also go some way to explaining the bizarre response of the food industry to these depressing statistics, which has in many cases been to place the blame on poor kitchen hygiene in the home. Although there can be no justification for the failure of the industry to put its own house in order, it is nevertheless true that foods that are 'free from preservatives' (including many special baby foods) are probably at greater risk of cross-contamination from other foods in the home, and do require particularly careful handling. We shall be discussing kitchen hygiene at the end of this chapter.

The surest way to avoid the harmful effects of food adulteration is of course to avoid altogether the foods which are most likely to be most highly adulterated. This means avoiding highly processed foods of all kinds, and whenever possible purchasing and preparing fresh, whole foods. Although this is true in general terms, it applies particularly to all foods and drinks consumed by young children, especially those under the age of five.

Whole Foods

By whole foods we mean those foods which have not been refined, or processed more than is necessary to render them edible; which have had nothing either added to or taken away from them.

The dangers to health from a loss of nutrients through refinement is particularly acute in relation to staple cereal foods. The basic diets of the vast majority of the peoples of the world have throughout history consisted of a single, 'staple', carbohydrate (usually a cereal such as wheat, maize, or rice),

---

* ibid., p. 238.

complemented and made palatable by small quantities of vegetables, fruits and meats, as these were available. This pattern has been radically altered over the last two or three hundred years in the affluent West, and two dietary changes in particular are now generally agreed to have been responsible, at least in part, for the marked increase (in the Western world) in the incidence of degenerative diseases of all kinds. These changes are: firstly, the shift in the balance of the general diet away from the 'core' starches and towards the richer 'supplementary' foods, meat in particular, with a huge increase in the consumption of fats and sugars; and secondly, and perhaps more damaging still, the increased refinement of the staple starch or carbohydrate foods themselves. In the UK, the introduction of new milling technology in the second half of the nineteenth century precipitated the almost total displacement of wholemeal bread by the nutritionally inferior bread made from refined white flour.

The nutritional disadvantages of a heavy reliance on refined carbohydrates are more widely understood now than they were a few years ago, but the recent resurgence in sales of white bread under the guise of supposedly healthy, supposedly fibre-rich, 'soft-grain' bread (supported by advertising campaigns specifically targeted at children) suggests that it may be worth rehearsing the main points briefly here. Wheat grains consist of three main elements: the starchy endosperm, which forms the bulk of the grain; the germ or embryo of the seed, which holds the grain's entire protein content and most of its vitamins; and the hard outer layers of bran, which are a valuable source of dietary fibre. Wholemeal flour retains all three parts in their natural proportions. The manufacture of white flour extracts and discards (or packages for sale as expensive 'health' foods) the germ and the bran, keeping only the starchy carbohydrate element of the grain. Wholemeal bread is a tasty, convenient and nutritious food, suitable for (and liked by) most children from the age of about six months onwards.

So much for the 'wholeness' of the whole foods we shall be recommending: what about the freshness? A series of chemical changes leading to eventual decomposition begins in most foods as soon as they are picked (or, in the case of animals and fish, killed). This deterioration progressively reduces the nutritional value of the food as vitamins and trace elements leach into the air, natural sugars are turned to starch, and fibrous cell walls break down.

A few whole foods are resistant to these processes. Most cereal grains, if stored away from moisture, light, and heat, remain fairly stable until milled, when a similar process of deterioration begins immediately. Dried pulses (the bean, pea and lentil family) and dried fruits, also have good storage qualities. But fresh fruits and vegetables, in particular, are *live* foods, and should be eaten as fresh as possible if they are to deliver in full their potential nutritional value. They should also be stored, prepared and cooked in such a way as to minimize the loss of nutrients. Most may in fact be eaten raw, and a proportion of raw food is an important element in a well-balanced diet. If cooked at all, it should be lightly: steaming is preferable to boiling for most vegetables.

The following list of foods, most of which are whole foods, is not intended to be exhaustive, but will give an idea of the kinds of ingredients that are used in the recipes in this book. Eating these foods yourself, and establishing a familiarity with them before the birth of your baby, will give you the confidence to experiment and adapt to the specific needs of your child later. And of course, as we have said already, it will be difficult for you to teach your child to enjoy foods which are very different from those you eat yourselves.

- Wholemeal flour, and wholemeal bread

- Whole cereal grains: rice, millet, wheat; also some white rice

- Cereal products: pasta and noodles, either white or wholewheat, cous-cous, rolled oats

- All fresh fruit and vegetables, as far as possible those in season, lightly cooked or eaten raw

- Dried beans and lentils

- Dried fruits, untreated if possible

- Eggs and dairy products: butter and cheese without colourings, plain, live yoghurt, milk or soya milk

■   Some meat, free-range or organically reared if possible, and some fish.

A variety of other foods may be used in addition to this basic list. Most people will want to use a selection of herbs and spices to add different flavours to their meals, though these should not be added to food that is to be given to young children. Lightly processed food products, such as tinned tomatoes and frozen peas, can also be used, although care should be taken – especially if they are to be used in children's food – to choose brands that are free from additives.

The best food for a baby from the day of its birth, and the only food it will need for the first few months of its life, is of course a whole food: its mother's milk. And, as we shall see, the quality of the mother's diet during pregnancy, and for as long as she breast-feeds, will affect the quality of her milk.

Organic Foods

The dangers associated with the adulteration of foodstuffs by the chemical residues of fertilizers and pesticides employed in modern agriculture cannot be sidestepped altogether simply by avoiding the use of processed foods. All the foods listed in the preceding section of this chapter may be contaminated in this way. Attention has recently been drawn, for example, to the widespread use on apples of Alar, banned in the USA where the official Environmental Protection Agency has said that there is an 'inescapable and direct correlation' between the use of the chemical and 'the development of life-threatening tumours'. Fresh fruits and vegetables should always be washed carefully before use, but poisonous chemical pesticides and fungicides, routinely sprayed on fresh produce, are frequently impossible to wash off. For children below the age of five, all non-organic fruit and vegetables and in particular potatoes, and any vegetables or fruits that are to be eaten raw, should always be peeled, so that toxic chemicals left on the skins will not be eaten.

'Organic' or 'organically grown' crops are produced and

stored without the use of dangerous chemicals, and provide one way of minimizing the risks of this kind of contamination. Children who show a tendency to allergic problems should certainly be kept as far as possible to an organic diet, and are very likely to show an improvement as a result. The snag is that organic produce, although it is increasingly widely available, still tends to be very much more expensive than its non-organic equivalent, and as long as demand (which is growing very fast at the moment) continues to outstrip supply, prices are likely to remain high.

Fresh organic fruits and vegetables, whether grown in your own garden or bought in a supermarket, certainly taste far better than ordinary ones, and there is considerable evidence that they are of superior nutritional value as well. Since they do not need to be peeled, the valuable vitamin and fibre content of the skins can also be retained. A compromise solution to the problem of price may be to concentrate on buying organic for important staple items such as bread, potatoes and brown rice, of which large quantities will be eaten, and where the price differential tends to be smallest. Anyone seeking further information on growing standards and sources of organic produce, or up-to-date news of developments in the movement, should contact the Soil Association, 86/88 Colston Street, Bristol, Avon BS1 5BB.

Sugar and Salt

Sugar and salt were both originally thought of as luxuries, but have become 'essentials'. They share the interesting characteristic that we find them easier to take up than to give up: as individuals and as nations we tend to consume ever-increasing quantities of both. Modern Western diets are dominated by these two flavouring substances to such an extent that they have come to define the most fundamental taste distinction made nowadays. And yet despite the importance of the perceived division of all tastes into the sweet and the savoury, the actual distinction is often blurred, and large quantities of both sugar *and* salt are used in the manufacture of many processed foods.

Sugar has come to be thought of as a food in itself, which it certainly is not. Sugars occur naturally in many fruits and vegetables, and as part of these whole foods they are nutritionally valuable, but sugar in its refined forms – either as the commonly used sucrose of packet sugars, or as glucose, dextrose, lactose, fructose, corn syrup, or any of the other sugars used in the manufacture of processed foods – can give us only 'empty' calories: it produces a passing surge of energy, but contains no lasting nourishment whatsoever.

Connections between the use of refined sugars and diabetes, heart disease and obesity have been widely researched but the evidence remains circumstantial so far. There is no doubt, however, about the role of sugar in tooth decay. The other obvious (and serious) danger of sugar, particularly for children, is that it tends to displace more nutritionally valuable foods in the diet. To the extent that a child's energy requirements are being met by his consumption of sugar, he will be correspondingly deprived of the proteins, vitamins and minerals which come packaged with the calories of whole, natural foods.

So all-pervasive has sugar become, that a belief has grown up that a liking for sugar is in itself natural, particularly among children (despite the fact that children constitute the group at greatest risk from sugar). Human milk is certainly sweet. But sugar itself has only been widely available in the West for about two hundred years, and even today it is used to very different extents by the peoples of various Western countries. The British are among the heaviest users.

... no ancestral predisposition within the species can adequately explain what are in fact culturally conventionalized norms, not biological imperatives ... On the one hand, that the human liking for sweetness is not just an acquired disposition is supported by many different kinds of evidence; on the other, the circumstances under which that predisposition is intensified by cultural practice are highly relevant to how strong the 'sweet tooth' is.*

Children do naturally like sweet things, but they do *not* have a natural craving for the intense sweetness of refined

---

* S. Mintz, *Sweetness and Power*, Penguin (1986), pp. 16–17.

sugar. Water, or very diluted fruit or vegetable juices, are perfectly adequate drinks for children from the time they first need other liquids in addition to breast (or bottle) milk, and are quite acceptable to most children. But a child's 'sweet tooth' is rapidly trained, and it will be difficult, if not impossible, to persuade a child to return to drinking water if he has already been taught to like sweet juices (whether artificially sweetened or not). A 'sweet tooth' soon turns into rotten teeth.

The same considerations apply to sweet foods. One instant dessert marketed for babies from the age of only three months contains maltodextrin, sucrose and dextrose. Other desserts are sweetened with concentrated fruit juices; as with drinks, their boast that they contain 'no added sugar' is no guarantee that they are not intensely sweet. 'Reduced sugar' infant rusks can contain around *20 per cent sugars* of one kind or another – sweeter than many ordinary biscuits and snacks for adults. Advertising campaigns specifically aimed at children encourage them to eat supposedly healthy foods such as, for instance, the Munch Bunch 'low fat' yoghurts. Flavours include 'Charlie' chocolate and 'Fergus' fudge ('Added ingredients: sugar, modified starch, flavouring').

Artificial sweeteners such as saccharin, cyclamate, aspartame (Nutrasweet), and Sunett are widely used as substitutes for sugar, especially in low-calorie drinks and foods. Foods and drinks containing any of these sweeteners should certainly not be given to children; there are doubts about the long-term safety of all of them (aspartame is particularly associated with hyperactivity in children), and they all act even more powerfully than sugar itself to hook children on sweetness.

Salt, on the other hand, which no one thinks of as a food in its own right, is actually essential, in small quantities, for many important bodily functions. The correct balance of salt in the body is maintained in healthy adults by the excretion of surpluses in sweat and urine, but a child's kidneys are unable to cope with large imbalances and can actually be damaged by excessive consumption of salt. Our advice will be to avoid the addition of salt to a child's food entirely. When you are going to blend, mash or chop some of the food you have cooked for the rest of the household, simply wait until you have extracted his portion before you add seasoning. The small quantities of salt he actually needs will easily be obtained from foods such as bread and cheese.

Meat

The reliance of the modern Western diet on meat as a major source of protein has, by a process similar to that which operates in relation to sugar, given rise to the widespread belief that regular daily consumption of some form of meat is a necessity for health from an early age. There are, however, many foods other than meat which are capable of supplying the necessary protein in a child's diet (see page 42). At the same time there are particular dangers associated with the eating of meat which, at least when choosing and preparing food for babies and young children, should be clearly understood and carefully weighed.

The first consideration is the delicate and still-developing digestive system of a young child. Just as a child is unable to chew adult food effectively until his first set of teeth is completely through when he is about two and a half years old, so his digestive system takes several years to acquire the bacterial and enzymic strength needed to break down many of the foods eaten by adults. Meat may be ground and puréed to enable a child to swallow it, but this does not mean that he will be able to digest it effectively.

Second, and more important, is the danger of meat and meat products as a source of food-poisoning, which has intensified over the last twenty or thirty years with the introduction of modern farming and food handling and processing practices. We often refer to our own upbringing as a guide, and may be inclined to say that 'I was given meat most days as a child and it never did me any harm.' With regard to meat at least, it is important for today's parents to recognize that things have changed significantly since they were children themselves.

The sheer numbers of animals that are raised together, often under one roof, in modern meat-rearing practice; the use of animal waste products such as bone and blood in the manufacture of the high-protein animal feeds used to fatten the animals; the routine use of antibiotics to promote growth and to treat disease, and the consequent development of resistant strains of infection; the multiplication of the opportunities for cross-contamination in modern production-line abattoirs; and the risk of meat being stored at the wrong temperature at some point in the extended distribution network from slaughterhouse to supermarket; all these factors lead to the conclusion that

It would be hard to devise a better, more efficient system of recycling salmonella than modern livestock farming. Its methods seem tailor-made to produce disease and spread infection amongst livestock destined for human consumption.*

And it is not only salmonella which is recycled. Bovine spongiform encephalitis (BSE), the fatal brain-rotting disease, which some doctors believe can be transmitted to humans from infected beef, is known to be contracted by cattle from feed containing protein recovered from the carcasses of sheep which were in turn infected with the associated scrapie disease.

Poultry – chicken and turkey – is probably easier for a child to digest than beef, lamb or pork, and is often given to children as their first meat. Unfortunately, of all meats poultry is the one most often implicated in the catalogue of risks outlined above. This is for two reasons: first, because – unlike cattle – infection with salmonella has no observable ill-effects on the live chickens, and therefore presents no incentive to the breeder to control the infection; and second, because chickens are very often frozen and then cooked as whole carcasses, with an increased risk that poor heat penetration into the interior of the bird will fail to destroy all contaminating micro-organisms.

The 'egg crisis' precipitated by Edwina Currie in December 1988 has been discussed in the Introduction to this book. What everyone now knows, thanks to the publicity she gave to the endemic salmonella infection in the UK poultry industry, is that *some* eggs carry salmonella; that the very young, the sick and the elderly are particularly at risk of contracting possibly

---

* London Food Commission, *Food Adulteration and How to Beat It* (1988), p. 245.

fatal food-poisoning from such eggs; and that only by boiling an egg for at least seven minutes can one be sure of killing any salmonella bacteria present in it.

Eggs have traditionally formed an important part of most children's diets. Will we now have to stop giving our children eggs altogether? We suggest the following guidelines as a sensible precautionary compromise. Assuming that the child shows no allergic reaction to eggs (see page 100), give eggs in moderation, but

■ not before nine months, and not if the child is poorly

■ well-boiled, not scrambled, poached or fried, and *never* raw

■ never give any food made with raw egg (mayonnaise, for example) unless you *know* the egg used was pasteurised.

Free-range eggs are produced humanely, but unfortunately the free-range label does not in itself guarantee that the hens have not been given feed concentrates containing recycled poultry carcasses. Eggs carrying the Soil Association symbol, however, are certified as having been produced organically, and certification includes a guarantee that no such feeds have been used.

There is no need to abstain from eating meat altogether, but when there is a baby or a young child in the household it is essential to be aware of the potential dangers, particularly from food-poisoning, whether or not he is to be given the meat himself. The greatest care must be taken to ensure not only that meat is thoroughly thawed if frozen, promptly and thoroughly cooked, and then immediately and quickly refrigerated if it is to be kept, but also that at every stage it is handled in such a way as to prevent the cross-contamination of other foods. Food-poisoning is of course extremely dangerous in young children, but even a fairly minor stomach upset early on, whether brought about by actual contamination or simply by eating over-rich and indigestible foods (which may include meat), can have a seriously disruptive effect on the development of healthy eating patterns and a settled digestive rhythm for months or even years to come.

Good cuts of lean meat are one thing, but 'meat products' should be avoided as far as possible. Sausages, pies and burgers, for example, may all contain chemical preservatives and poly-phosphates to increase the water retention of the meat. They may also contain meat from heads, tails and feet, and mechani-cally recovered meat (MRM), without any legal requirement to declare the proportions of non-lean meat used. MRM is col-lected from animal carcasses by stripping the bones of gristle, sinew and remaining shreds of meat to produce a paste of small meat particles. This is not only of lower nutritional value than lean meat, but it is also thought to be more likely to harbour bacteria. Free-range and organically produced meat can be found, and is not always as expensive as one might expect. Care must of course still be exercised in storing and handling, but it makes a pleasant change to eat meat which one knows to be free of drug residues, free of BSE, and to come from an animal which has been humanely raised. As with eggs, Soil Association organic certification guarantees that animals have not been given feeds containing recycled animal carcasses.

Special Diets and Allergies

The primary meaning of the word 'diet' is simply 'that which is eaten' by an individual or a group. This book contains advice and recipes for parents wishing to bring up a child using any one of three general diets, all of them based on the use of whole (as opposed to processed) foods: a *mixed* diet, including some meat and fish; a *vegetarian* diet, excluding meat and fish, but including animal products such as eggs and cheese; and a *vegan* diet, excluding all animal products.

The choice between these three ways of eating is a matter of preference, and there are advantages and disadvantages to each. Meat provides an excellent and simple source of protein, but, as explained above, we do not recommend giving it to a child under the age of twelve months. Even after this age, meat should be introduced very gradually and with great care, bearing in mind the possibility of an adverse reaction. A completely vegetarian or vegan household avoids the risks of food-poisoning that are associated with meat, and will be saved the extra precautions which must be taken wherever meat is used (whether or not it is to be given to a child); in addition, there will be a cost saving in comparison with a diet that includes meat and meat products (which might be used to pay the premiums on organically grown fruit and vegetables). A vegan diet specifically excludes the animal products which are the most straightforward source of complete proteins, and attention needs to be paid to combining food ingredients correctly so as to avoid protein deficiency, which is especially dangerous for growing children (see page 42), and to ensuring a sufficient intake of calcium and vitamin B_{12} (see page 45).

A secondary meaning of the word 'diet', 'a prescribed course of food, restricted in kind or quantity', has quite recently overtaken the original meaning in day-to-day usage. Modern diets of this kind are almost always designed, at least in part, to achieve a measurable goal of weight gain or (more often) weight loss. They very often have the unintended effect of aggravating that breakdown of response between appetite and bodily needs which is commonly the root cause of the very problem the diet was intended to alleviate. It is for this reason, for example, that slimmers find it so difficult to maintain the weight loss achieved in the first few months of dieting.

Diets of this kind, whether for weight loss or weight gain, whether low fat or high fibre, should *never* be used for a growing child unless under the strict instructions of a qualified practitioner. Parents who themselves follow special diets no doubt do so because they believe it is good for them, and must take particular care to avoid making the assumption that what is good for them is also good for their child.

A mother who is deeply concerned about maintaining her own slim figure may find that she feels embarrassed by the roly-poly chubbiness of her six-month-old baby. A father may want his toddler to become a big strapping child to compensate for his own feeling of weakness, or to demonstrate his ability to provide well for his child. But as long as the natural integration of a child's eating with his physical needs is not broken down, his body will control its own growth for optimum health, and fluctuations in body-weight should not be interfered with. Most particularly, no attempt should ever be made to *reduce* a child's weight, even if it is above the average for his age.

Certain foods may have to be avoided by an individual child because they have been found to cause allergic reactions. Most children will never suffer in this way, but parents should be aware of the possibility that their child may develop allergies and should be prepared to notice the symptoms as soon as they occur, especially if there is a history of allergies in a member of their close family. It is worth trying to remember or find out whether you or your partner, or any of your child's grandparents, suffered as children from allergies of any kind, particularly asthma or eczema. Most children who suffer in this way eventually grow out of their allergies (which is why you may be unaware that a close relative ever had such a problem), but while the allergies last they must not be ignored even when the symptoms they produce are fairly minor.

Allergies occur when the body reacts to a substance as if it were harmful. The allergic symptoms themselves are a secondary consequence of this response. By no means all allergies are food-related, but those that are can result in a range of allergic symptoms of widely varying severity, from rashes to eczema and asthma. One of the most troublesome food allergies, known as coeliac disease, results from an intolerance of gluten, which is a natural protein found in the starchy part of some cereal grains. It is present in the largest quantities in wheat, and is the element of wheat flour which enables us to bake leavened bread. Gluten is present in smaller quantities in rye, and to a lesser extent still in barley and oats. Millet, rice and maize, as well as the non-cereal flours made from buckwheat and soya, are entirely gluten-free. We recommend the use of only gluten-free cereals up to the age of six months, when barley and oats, and then wheat, can be slowly and carefully introduced. Remember that many common foods other than bread, and especially many manufactured foods (such as sausages, for example), contain wheat or derivatives of wheat. Further details on allergies are given in Chapter 4 (see page 100).

Susceptibility to allergies fluctuates both in children and in adults in relation to background levels of stress. The types of stress which appear to erode resistance to allergies (particularly in children) include psychological strain, illness, fatigue, disruption of routine, other allergies, and all 'foreign' substances, by which we mean the huge number of chemicals now present in our air and water as well as in our food. A child who has a cold may react violently to a food which he has happily eaten when he was well. Conversely, reducing the stress load in any of the areas we have mentioned may enable a child to tolerate foods which otherwise act as allergens. Nor are allergies always absolute: a child may be able to eat small amounts of a food allergen without a reaction. A completely organic, additive-free diet (see page 32), and the use of purified water (see page 46), are often found to help greatly by raising the level of tolerance.

Proteins, Carbohydrates, Fats, Vitamins and Minerals

A basic understanding of the various constituent elements of a well-balanced diet and an awareness of the significance of a few key vitamins will normally be enough to enable parents to provide their child with a healthy diet, and to do so with confidence. The human race would not have survived into the twentieth century if a thorough grounding in nutritional science was an indispensable prerequisite of successful parenthood. A child who eats a well-balanced diet of unprocessed foods is unlikely ever to run the slightest risk of a deficiency of any essential nutrient.

Protein is the basic building material of the body, and is essential for growth and for healing. It is therefore particularly important to ensure sufficient protein in the diet of a child. Many foods provide protein, but not all can supply *by themselves* the 'complete protein' specifically required by the human body. Meat, fish, eggs, cheese, and other dairy products, are single foods which are all sources of complete protein. Other foods are excellent sources of 'incomplete' or 'near-complete' protein, and must be eaten *in combination* (in other words, together and at the same time) if the body is to derive from them the complete protein it needs.

A small amount of cow's milk or cheese completes the

protein content of cereals such as wheat, rice and millet, and of some vegetables such as potatoes. Combinations giving complete protein which do not involve the use of any animal products include cereals with pulses (rice and peas or beans, for example) and pulses with sesame, pumpkin or sunflower seeds. Tahini, the semi-liquid paste made by grinding sesame seeds, complements many incomplete protein foods as well as being nutritious in its own right, and adds body and flavour to almost any meal for a child. Soya beans are well known as a rich source of near-complete protein. They are neither as easy to use nor as tasty as other beans in their whole state, but soya bean curd (or tofu) is especially useful for children on diets which exclude meat.

A lack of protein in the diet is not the only possible cause of protein deficiency. Carbohydrates provide the body with its energy (or calories), and if insufficient carbohydrates are consumed the body is forced to burn off protein to supply the energy it needs. The human species has evolved as eaters of large quantities of carbohydrates, and it is only recently, and only in the affluent West, that the balance of the common diet has shifted away from this core of starch towards the richer, higher-protein foods which the majority of the world's population still thinks of as supplementary to their basic staple.

It is necessary to distinguish between the *complex* carbohydrates of whole cereal grains and their products (and of other starchy foods such as potato and cassava) and the *simple* carbohydrate of sugar. As described above in relation to wheat (see page 30), unrefined complex carbohydrate foods not only deliver large quantities of the starches which the body burns as calories, but carry with them a valuable supply of fibre, protein and vitamins. Sugars, on the other hand, are simple carbohydrates, and even unrefined sugar is almost totally devoid of any additional nutrients.

In the literal sense of the word, the 'bulk' of a child's diet from the time he starts to take solids should be made up of unrefined complex carbohydrates. Wholemeal bread, brown rice, millet, oats, wholewheat breakfast cereal, pasta, potatoes and other similar foods provide a healthy staple basis for any diet. There is nothing at all wrong with the old-fashioned habit of basing each day's main meals around a different starchy food, ending up with roast potatoes for Sunday lunch! If the majority of the starches are provided in unrefined form, they will (together with the other foods given) supply the child with all the protein, calories, fibre, vitamins and minerals he needs. He will develop strong bones and teeth, his digestion will be settled and efficient, his eyes and skin clear, and he will have the strength to combat infection and disease effectively.

Tiny quantities of certain fats are essential for specific physical functions, and certain fats are the only sources of important 'fat soluble' vitamins. But it would be difficult to go short of these fats while eating any kind of balanced diet, and an excess of fats of all kinds is far more common. Fats are the most concentrated source of calories, which is why the consumption of fried foods is likely to cause problems of overweight. It is sensible to keep the amount of fried food in a child's diet to an absolute minimum. It is also important to use unrefined cold-pressed vegetable oils whenever possible rather than the so-called 'pure' refined cooking oils, which are produced using a variety of heat and chemical treatments to maximize the yield and to deodorize, bleach and stabilize the oil. In many of them the fats become saturated (and therefore of reduced nutritional value) in the course of the refining process.

As long as a baby is either breast-feeding or taking formula milk from a bottle as its principal source of nourishment, there should be no danger of vitamin or mineral deficiencies. Depending on the mixture of foods introduced as the child makes the transition to solid foods, a shortfall of certain vitamins may occur briefly at this stage, particularly if the child is weaned early, and many doctors recommend the use of vitamin drops as a precautionary measure for all children for a few months after weaning. Vitamin C, which helps the body fight off infection and which aids the absorption of iron, cannot be stored by the body. Both of these properties are especially important for children, so make sure that your child gets a regular supply of those foods which contain vitamin C. Citrus fruit is the best source; lightly cooked green vegetables, and bean sprouts, are also good sources.

For children on diets which exclude all animal products,

care must be taken to include sources of sufficient calcium and vitamin B_{12} in the diet. Good sources of calcium include: sesame seeds and tahini, seaweeds, and brewer's yeast (in powdered or flaked form) which is also rich in other minerals. Vitamin B_{12} is contained in seaweeds and in fermented soya bean paste (or miso); if neither of these sources is used, a supplementary source of this vitamin should probably be taken.

Recipes, Equipment, Storage and Hygiene

Delicious, varied and nutritious meals can be prepared from fresh, whole ingredients without fuss or anxiety, and without the need to follow precise recipes. No one with a small child wants to spend their life in the kitchen, and our aim is to provide suggestions, methods and recipes that will enable parents to give an excellent diet without requiring them to spend more than about an hour a day (on average) preparing food. Flexibility is an important factor where children are concerned, and recipes that call for pinpoint accuracy either in timing or in quantities will be excluded. Let soufflés wait till your children are older; in the meantime it will be better to stick to dishes which can easily be adapted to make use of the ingredients that are ready to hand, and which will not be ruined if the mealtime is delayed for fifteen minutes.

The detailed recommendations for methods of food preparation contained in the chapters that follow this one, and the specific recipes at the end of the book, will assume that you have the following basic items of equipment:

Stove (gas or electric) with grill and oven

Refrigerator with freezer compartment

Electric kettle

Electric blender

2 good-sized saucepans (preferably stainless steel)

Smaller saucepan (stainless steel) specifically for the baby

Large cast-iron frying pan

Good-sized casserole (preferably suitable for stove top as well as oven)

Chopping-board for vegetables

Small chopping-board for meat and fish (if these are to be used)

2 good sharp knives, one large, one small

Wooden spoon

Wooden spatula

Flexible spatula (plastic rather than rubber)

For your child:

Plastic bowl

6 small plastic spoons

6 10 fl oz (½ pt) plastic containers with sealing tops for freezing meal-sized portions (up to about twelve months)

'Teacher beaker' (either without handles or with two, but *not* with one; preferably with a sealing travelling top)

and if required:

5 fl oz (¼ pt) bottle

10 fl oz (½ pt) bottle

2 teats of colourless silicone (not yellow latex), preferably with a valve to prevent a vacuum forming in the bottle as the baby sucks

Bottle brush

More equipment will be needed for full bottle-feeding (see page 79).

A freezer is useful but by no means essential; a hand blender is useful to purée one meal in the bowl, and is easy to clean, but a jug-type blender is preferable so that at least three meals can be prepared at the same time: the cheaper models are perfectly adequate despite having only one speed and no other attachments, the only drawback being that the blades are generally not removable and therefore require particular care when they are washed. A tin-opener, a garlic-press, a lemon-squeezer, an apple-corer, a vegetable-steamer and a water-filter are all useful and inexpensive additions to the basic list above.

Water-filters remove from tap water a significant proportion of both mineral and bacterial contaminants, including traces of lead from old water pipes. They also remove most of the chemicals added to mains water as purifying agents, and (in hard water areas) much of the lime which leads to the formation of scale in kettles and pans. The most common and convenient water-filter is the jug type, with an upper half that is filled from the kitchen tap, and a lower half to collect the filtered water. Whatever kind is used, it is essential to change the filter cartridge at regular intervals (usually of about a month, but depending on water consumption), to prevent the build-up of contaminants filtered out of the water from reaching levels at which they might spill back into it in quantities even larger than normal.

Storage is an important element in organizing food for minimum inconvenience and maximum flexibility. As long as a young child still requires food which is different from yours, a great deal of time can be saved by preparing three or four portions for freezing in addition to the one that will be eaten immediately. A good supply of a range of dry ingredients, properly stored, ensures that there will always be food in the home even when you have run out of meals prepared in advance, and on those occasions when it proves impossible to get to the shops.

Fresh fruit and vegetables should be purchased at least weekly, and most vegetables benefit from being stored in the refrigerator till used. The exceptions are onions and garlic; potatoes and carrots (both of which keep best if they are bought unwashed and only scrubbed immediately before use); celery (which should be kept in water but away from light); and mustard and cress (which should be left in its punnet by a window and kept moist). Cereal grains and flours, dried pulses (lentils and beans), nuts, seeds and dried fruit should all be kept in airtight jars away from heat and direct light.

Meals that are prepared in advance should be cooled as rapidly as possible once they are made, then sealed in clean containers and put in the freezer immediately. The freezing compartment of an ordinary domestic refrigerator should be able to cope with three or even four 10 fl oz pots of food at a time in this way, though it will need to be turned up a little from its normal setting in order to maintain the temperature of 5°C required for effective refrigeration. Frozen meals must be thoroughly reheated before serving; stir to eliminate 'cold spots' in the pot. Food that has once been frozen and thawed must be thrown out if not used at once. *Even vegetarian meals must never be refrozen and reheated.*

Keep your refrigerator defrosted and clean. All food should be carefully sealed to prevent cross-contamination, and in particular raw and cooked food should be kept apart. It is especially important that, if meat is used, it is not allowed to come into contact with other foods, either in the refrigerator or elsewhere, and a separate chopping-board (preferably of hard plastic) should always be used for cutting meat of any kind.

Always wash your hands thoroughly both before preparing food for your child and before feeding him, and once he is crawling wash his hands before every meal too. A kitchen hand-towel should be kept carefully distinct from any cloth or towel used to dry pots and dishes. One cloth (which can be replaced or put in the wash once a week) should be kept exclusively for wiping your child after his meal. Ordinary kitchen cloths are made in several colours; you can reserve one colour exclusively for your child's face and hands. Once he starts to eat solids you will probably need to wipe the floor several times a day. *Never* use either the child's face-cloth or the washing-up/wiping-down cloth to mop the floor. Keep a special floor-cloth somewhere near to hand, and away from food.

2 Diet for Pregnancy and Labour

Eating for Two

The intensity and the intimacy of pregnancy, as of childbirth itself, are not easily accepted by the 'normal' world of everyday social contacts, and generalized concepts (often couched in humorous terms) are one way in which the everyday world seeks to protect itself from the disturbing, elemental quality of this most natural of events. So 'You're eating for two' often becomes a jocular encouragement to a pregnant woman to use her pregnancy as an excuse for over-indulgence; the importance of the pregnancy itself is thus played down, and the woman ransomed from the dangerous realm of blood and instinct into the comfortable commonplace.

Of course it is true in a physical sense that from the moment of conception until she stops breast-feeding a mother is indeed eating for two. While breast-feeding, she will actually need to eat more to supply the extra calories required for milk production. This is not the case during pregnancy, but the developing foetus is nevertheless fed by her blood passing through the placenta, and all its nourishment is ultimately derived from the food which the mother consumes. We will consider the pregnant mother's nutritional requirements later in the chapter.

But the knowledge that she is eating not only for herself but for her child is also a key element in a mother's preparation for bearing and caring for her baby. It gives her the opportunity, in the long months of pregnancy, to accustom herself to the often conflicting feelings aroused in her by the dependence of her child on her care and her nurturing. Both from a nutritional and from an emotional point of view, the earlier a couple start to care for their child in this way the better. Problems of infertility which haved failed to respond to any of the treatments available may sometimes be overcome by a change of diet. Not only will a healthy diet for both partners give them the best possible chance of conceiving, but – just as important – it will concentrate their minds on practical efforts to 'make space' for the child they want.

Research into pre-conceptual care suggests that the quality of both mother's and father's diet in the months prior to conception can have an effect on the health of the foetus. Diet in this sense must include the use of alcohol, coffee, cigarettes, and other drugs including both prescribed and over-the-counter types (see page 57). There is another reason why the introduction of healthy eating habits *before* the planned conception takes place is so widely recommended. This is of course the fact that, even with modern pregnancy testing techniques, it is impossible to know that a baby has been conceived until it is two weeks old at the absolute earliest. From the first days of pregnancy foetal development crucially depends on the health of the mother, and heart, nervous system, brain and spinal cord all begin to form in the early weeks. Poor diet is also widely accepted as one among many factors which may affect the chances of miscarriage.

Eating Well

As noted in the previous chapter, pregnancy presents the opportunity for a nine-month-long reappraisal and adjustment of what you eat, and the way in which you prepare and eat it. This is the time to establish not just a well-balanced diet, but a well-balanced attitude to food as well. Changes made now will produce multiple benefits: they will aid the development of the foetus, improving the chances that your baby will be born strong and healthy; they will tone and strengthen your own body, increasing your resilience to withstand the rigours of labour and the demands of breast-feeding; and they will lay the foundations for a simple and flexible routine for the preparation of enjoyable and nourishing family meals.

If you decide on major changes in the type of food you eat, you should make these changes over a period of months rather than all at once. Your body will take time to adjust to a change of diet, even when this is an improvement on what it has been used to. New ingredients will require new preparation techniques, and these will also take a little time to get used to; introduce new foods gradually, in a way which does not jeopardize your enjoyment of either the preparation or the eating of your meals.

The most beneficial overall changes that you can make are to cut down on sugar and foods sweetened with sugar, and to shift the balance of your diet away from processed foods (whether in packets or tins bought from the supermarket for heating and eating at home, or of the ready-to-eat, fast-food variety) and towards the use of fresh, whole foods. You may feel that pregnancy is a time for the conservation of energy, and that the last thing you will feel like doing is to spend time preparing complicated meals. In fact, the unhurried, methodical preparation of a delicious meal, with your thoughts centred on the baby growing in your womb and on the nourishment and satisfaction you and she will both derive from it, can be a delightful meditation for pregnancy. If you are tired or hurried, however, there are plenty of ways of cooking healthy meals from fresh ingredients without much more effort than it would take to make up a mug of packet soup; and the better your diet during pregnancy, the more energy you will have and the less tired you are likely to feel.

The following tips are all of general application, but apply particularly during pregnancy:

Share the work Partners should share (to some extent at least) the work involved in *all* aspects of the cycle of family feeding, from shopping to chopping, and from dishing up to washing up.

Keep it simple Keep things simple; good fresh ingredients do not need to be disguised beneath complicated sauces. There is no point in making two courses if doing so leaves you so exhausted or so resentful that you are unable to take pleasure in eating them; make a main dish and follow it with fruit.

Quantities Prepare food in sufficient quantities either to freeze half for use later or at least to leave leftovers for heating up the next day. Follow the basic rules for the storage of cooked food (see page 47).

Tidiness Keep the kitchen tidy. Cooking a meal takes far longer, and is far more stressful, if you have to spend time looking for every ingredient and every piece of equipment, or if each cooking session has to start with half an hour's tidying up in order to clear a space to work in.

Comfort Organize the kitchen for maximum comfort. Many jobs can be done sitting down if there is a chair or stool and a work surface of the right height. A work surface with room underneath it for your knees is a help, but a kitchen table will often serve just as well. If possible, hang the most regularly used pans and utensils where they can be reached without bending (this will also be useful when your child starts to crawl and stand). Bad lighting puts a strain on your eyes and tends to make you stoop over your work, and can lead to accidents and poor kitchen hygiene.

The quality of a mother's diet during pregnancy will affect not only the development of the baby in her womb, but also her own health and vitality, and the amount and quality of the milk she produces when the baby is born. From conception onwards foetal development takes priority over a mother's own needs in the way her body allocates its resources. One third of the mother's reserves of iron, for example, are typically employed in the formation of foetal blood. The foetus will take from her body what it requires in the way of nutrients, provided that what it requires is available, and it will do this in some cases even at the expense of the mother's health.

The general rules for a good diet apply in pregnancy as at any other time. It should be based around a variety of unrefined carbohydrate foods (whole grain cereals and wholemeal bread), and should include adequate complete protein derived from meat and/or from a combination of vegetable foods. Adjustments to a healthy, well-balanced diet may be made in order to relieve symptoms of flatulence, nausea, indigestion, or constipation (see page 55), but these must be tailored to individual cases. There are very few modifications which can be recommended in general terms, but calcium deficiency, anaemia and high blood pressure are common complaints of pregnancy, and can all be mitigated by adjustments to the diet.

Calcium deficiency is the result of the draining of reserves of calcium to meet the needs of the growing baby as it forms bones and teeth. It can result in brittle nails, hair loss, and tooth decay in the mother, and is likely to cause painful cramps in her calf muscles. All fresh vegetables and to a lesser extent all fresh fruits contain calcium. Other foods particularly rich in calcium include: cheddar cheese, molasses, brewer's yeast, beans, sesame and sunflower seeds, and seaweeds.

Anaemia is associated with a deficiency of iron in the diet, and is commonly treated in pregnancy with iron supplements. These have the unfortunate side-effect in some women, however, of increasing the tendency to constipation which many pregnant women suffer anyway. Increasing the proportion of iron-rich foods in the diet can provide a solution. These include: red meat (especially liver), eggs, pumpkin and sesame seeds, molasses, brewer's yeast, soya beans, wholemeal bread, and (among vegetables) parsley, broccoli and radishes. A good regular supply of vitamin C greatly assists the efficient absorption of iron.

Brewer's yeast, which appears in both these lists, and is also one of the best available sources of B-vitamins, is a by-product of beer production and not, as the name seems to suggest, the yeast used by brewers to begin the fermentation of the beer. It can be bought from health food shops, and comes in two forms: as a brown powder, and as small yellow-brown yeast flakes, which are more palatable to some people but very much more expensive. In either form, brewer's yeast should be added in small amounts to soups and stews just before they are served, or sprinkled on to individual servings.

There is some evidence that high blood pressure is helped by a reduction in the consumption of red meat and of salt and salty foods, and excessive salt in the diet also tends to exacerbate problems of fluid retention (see page 57). If there is a particular risk of miscarriage, you may wish to increase your intake of folic acid, which is now thought to be significant in the prevention of repeated miscarriages when taken both in the months prior to conception and in the early months of pregnancy. Good sources of folic acid include: black-eye beans, spinach, wholemeal bread, oranges, eggs and (once again) brewer's yeast.

Weight Gain

Weight gain is a natural and necessary part of pregnancy. In addition to the weight of the growing child itself, the mother's body lays down reserves which will be called on for the production of breast milk after the baby is born. This is a quite involuntary process, and cannot be prevented without risk to the healthy development of the unborn child, even if the mother has already decided that she is not going to breast-feed. (On the other hand, of course, it will be much harder to lose the extra weight after the baby is born if she is not breast-feeding.)

As we have seen, body weight is a focus of almost universal neurosis in our modern culture; obesity is a widespread problem, due to our sedentary lifestyle and our unhealthy diet, while at the same time we idolize, particularly in women, the ultra-slim figure which is simply unattainable for most of us once we have passed puberty. Weight gain can be a problem in pregnancy, but it is much less commonly a physical problem than it is a psychological one, and partners and friends have an important supportive role to play in reassuring a pregnant woman that she has not lost any of her charm. The presence of a pregnant woman who is able to enjoy her changing body shape with pride and satisfaction can be powerfully attractive.

Weight gain during pregnancy varies widely from woman to woman, but will not exceed what your body demands as a natural part of its preparation for motherhood if you limit your consumption of sugar, exclude deep-fried foods, and cut down (but do not cut out) your consumption of other fatty foods such as meat and dairy products.

Food cravings are enshrined in folklore as an essential element of every pregnancy. They are a remarkable instance of the human body's ability to stimulate a conscious appetite for the foods it needs, which is noticeable as a phenomenon particular to pregnant women because the rapidly changing needs of their bodies trigger new appetites. They may take a variety of forms, and for the most part should be attended to, as they are likely to arise from a genuine bodily need. Try to satisfy the cravings in a healthy way, however: choose fruits rather than chocolate to satisfy a taste for sweetness, for instance.

Attempts to limit weight gain unduly will of course result in food cravings of a rather different kind as the increased calorific requirements of the body make themselves felt in acute hunger. But as long as the bulk of the carbohydrate content of the diet is unrefined – coming from wholemeal bread, brown rice and potatoes, for example – there is no reason to worry that an increased intake of carbohydrates will lead to excessive weight gain. The unrefined carbohydrates of whole foods will satisfy hunger for a longer period, will tone the digestion to ease constipation and aid the absorption of nutrients, and are less likely to lay down superfluous fatty tissue.

Sickness and Indigestion

Some women experience considerable digestive discomfort during pregnancy. Typically, symptoms of nausea are worst on waking and through the first part of the day (hence 'morning sickness') and pass or diminish after the first three months of the pregnancy, although this pattern is by no means universal.

Adjustment of diet and eating patterns often provides an effective way of treating morning sickness. Various general points are worth observing:

Fatty foods   Fatty foods such as milk, butter and cheese, as well as deep-fried food, generally make the symptoms worse. Cut down on these and replace the calcium supplied by dairy products with calcium-rich vegetable foods (see page 53).

Protein   An imbalance in the proportion of protein to carbohydrate in the diet is likely to make the symptoms worse. In pregnancy, as at other times, *at least* two parts (by cooked volume) of carbohydrate foods should be eaten to every one part of protein-rich food. Cut down on meat and meat products, and increase consumption of wholemeal bread and whole cooked cereal grains.

Mealtimes   Be flexible about your mealtimes. Five or six small meals a day may be easier for your digestive system to deal with than two heavy ones, and if you are unable to eat enough to keep you going at normal mealtimes it is better to increase the number of proper meals than to snack on biscuits and chocolate bars. Make sure that each of your meals is healthy and balanced, particularly with regard to the formation of complete protein (see page 42). You can simply take your main meal of the day in two instalments, but if it consists of salad and stew, for instance, have some salad and some stew at each serving. Some women find that morning sickness is relieved by eating something before they get up in the morning. Try leaving an apple and a slice of plain bread or a couple of unsweetened biscuits beside your bed the night before.

Following these suggestions will probably make you more comfortable throughout pregnancy, whether or not you suffer from actual morning sickness. In addition to the hormonal changes occurring in your body and the new demands made on your digestive system by the baby, as she grows your stomach will be pushed up into the body cavity by the top of your womb. This in itself is likely to make it uncomfortable to eat much at a sitting, so the advice to eat little and often is certainly helpful to most mothers.

Every individual is different, and it is important to pay attention to the possible connections between particular foods and the worsening of indigestion or nausea. Cut out the worst-offending foods, at least for a couple of weeks, but be sure not to unbalance your diet by doing so: substitute vegetable for vegetable, carbohydrate for carbohydrate, and protein for protein. Do not take indigestion remedies without reference to a qualified practitioner.

In general, you should expect a slight slowing down of your digestive system during pregnancy, but this should not lead to discomfort as long as most of the food in your diet is unrefined. Constipation may be made worse by taking iron supplements. Try to avoid the necessity of taking supplements by making sure you eat plenty of iron-rich foods (see page 53). Raw fruit and vegetables provide bulk and fibre which will ease constipation, as well as being a valuable source of vitamins, and it may be a good idea to base your midday meal on raw vegetables.

Fluid retention is a common complaint, particularly in the later stages of pregnancy, and leads to uncomfortable swollen ankles and sore feet. Fluid retention is related to blood pressure, and will be regularly monitored as part of your ante-natal care. It is a normal part of pregnancy and swelling usually disappears very soon after the baby is born. Limiting the amount of salt in the diet is likely to help, but do not attempt to control fluid retention by cutting down your intake of liquids. Eat plenty of fresh fruits and vegetables, and try to take regular short breaks through the day to relax with your feet level with your body. Blackberry-leaf tea also helps to relieve the symptoms of fluid retention.

Some of the suggestions we have made may present problems for women who choose to continue working during their pregnancy. They may be expected to rely on a sandwich bar or staff canteen for food throughout the day, and may find it difficult to take food breaks when they need to do so. Tell your work colleagues of your pregnancy as soon as it begins to affect the way you feel, and share your feelings with them openly. Notify employer and union representative, too. Do not make unreasonable requests, but make it clear that you expect some allowance to be made for your condition. Eat little and often if you can, but make sure that what you eat each time is healthy and satisfying. *Always* make time to sit down and relax when you eat. A staff canteen may be able to make special arrangements to suit you. Your pregnancy may be a trivial event from the perspective of the business you work for, but from the point of view of your baby it is unique and all-important. You have a responsibility to care for her, and a right to expect that others will assist you to do so.

Alcohol, Cigarettes, Caffeine and Medicines

From the moment of conception, a mother is not only eating for two but drinking and smoking for two as well. Both alcohol and cigarettes are known to affect the development of the foetus, and both have proven associations with miscarriage. Alcohol passes through the placenta into the baby's system, and should be kept to the occasional and *moderate* consumption of drinks other than spirits. Smoking during pregnancy reduces the amount of oxygen in the mother's bloodstream that is available to her child, and is known to lead to small babies with an increased vulnerability to infections. Caffeine (in tea as well as in coffee) is a powerful stimulant, and should be used in moderation. It is not known whether caffeine directly affects the foetus, but it certainly enters the mother's bloodstream, and it inhibits her absorption of iron, which as we have seen is an important nutrient during pregnancy. Medicines and drugs, of whatever kind, should be taken only after consultation with a qualified practitioner.

For some women, social pressure to continue drinking alcohol will be more difficult to resist during pregnancy than their own inclination to do so. Good friends will, however, understand and respect your wishes. They will, in the same way, refrain from smoking right beside you. Secondary smoking is known to affect foetal development, and you need not hesitate to ask people not to envelop you in cigarette smoke.

Cups of tea and coffee are the stepping-stones of mental as well as physical refreshment by which many of us pick our path through the day. Caffeine-free herbal teas are much more widely available than they used to be, often in tea-bag form, and provide a variety of refreshing alternatives to the pick-me-ups of coffee and tea. Try to substitute herbal teas for some, if not all, of the hot drinks of the day, especially in the second half of the day: you should sleep better as a result, and will therefore be less likely to feel the need of strong tea or coffee to get you going in the morning. Japanese twig (or bancha) tea is a low-caffeine product from the same bush that produces ordinary tea-leaves, and is an extremely rich source of calcium which makes it an ideal alternative to regular tea during pregnancy. It can be found in good wholefood or health food shops. Useful herbal teas (some of which can now be found in ordinary supermarkets) include: chamomile, which is a mild natural relaxant, aids digestion and makes a good night-time drink; rosehip, which has a refreshing fruity flavour and is rich in vitamin C; raspberry-leaf, which tones the muscles of the uterus in preparation for labour; and blackberry-leaf, which is a mild diuretic.

Homoeopathic remedies for minor illnesses are well worth considering as an alternative to ordinary medical drugs during pregnancy. Unlike ordinary medicines, which chemically alter the body's functions and which must all affect an unborn baby once they have entered her mother's bloodstream, homoeopathic remedies alert and mobilize the body's own defences, and have no known side-effects. Homoeopathy can also be effective in assisting the physical and psychological preparation for labour and the demands of motherhood. Do not attempt to prescribe your own remedies, however: if you wish to use homoeopathic treatments you should consult a qualified practitioner.

Food and Drink for Labour

Preparation for labour itself should also include some consideration of food and drink. At the onset of labour, try if you have time to eat a light, nutritious meal with plenty of calories for energy. It is probably a good idea to avoid meat of any kind at this time, but a couple of cheese sandwiches, buttered toast and a boiled egg, or (if you have some frozen or refrigerated) a bowl of thick vegetable soup with a slice of bread, would all be ideal. If, as often happens, fully established labour is delayed for more than a few hours, again eat a light, calorie-rich meal.

Once labour is established, with contractions coming at regular intervals, you ought not (and will probably not want) to eat at all. You will, however, need something to give you energy if labour is prolonged, so have a small jar of honey with you and take a teaspoonful every hour or so. You will probably feel very thirsty, but should avoid drinking more than an *occasional sip* of liquid. Have a bottle of spring water with you for this purpose. Sucking on an ice-cube also helps to relieve thirst, and having your face and lips wiped with a moistened cloth is refreshing.

The Bach flower Rescue Remedy is a useful general tonic which can be taken under the tongue from a dropper at intervals throughout labour, and if you use homoeopathic remedies, your homoeopath may be able to give you one to take during labour to help you keep on top of the pain and the fear. These options share the advantage that they will not conflict with any of the medical drugs which may be offered by the midwife and which you may choose to take as well.

If you are going to have the baby in hospital, you may like to take your own herbal teas, spring water and fresh fruit with you, and perhaps a loaf of wholemeal bread. If you have a prolonged stay in hospital, make sure that you maintain the standard of your normal diet as nearly as you can. If necessary, ask your partner or friends to bring special foods to supplement or replace what the hospital provides.

3 Breast-feeding and Bottle-feeding

Breast or Bottle?

Moments after the umbilical cord is cut and the baby is put to her breast, his mother continues to feed him, not now with her blood but with her milk. Lactation is a spontaneous physiological process set in motion by the action of the baby's sucking, and the milk that his mother produces is as complete a food for him as the blood that flowed from her body through the placenta, perfectly tailored to meet his individual nutritional needs. The physical and psychological union of mother and baby which begins with conception and continues through pregnancy to birth is completed by breast-feeding, which at the same time introduces the baby to the external world of sensation, taste, smell, sight and sound at a pace which matches his own unique rate of development.

Only since the introduction of modern techniques of pasteurization, hygienic storage and drying of cow's milk has there been any alternative to breast-feeding. These technical advances enabled doctors in the 1940s and 1950s to propound 'scientific' feeding routines based on measured quantities of formula milk given from the bottle. Over the course of the last century women have found their understanding of and responsibility for their own and their children's health and welfare eroded, as control has passed out of their hands and into those of the medical professionals; the widespread acceptance of 'scientific' feeding paralleled the general medicalization of obstetric care, from conception through pregnancy and birth.

The belief grew up that breast-fed babies were undernourished. When culturally accepted science imposes on a mother its 'expert knowledge' of what is best for the healthy development of her baby, she is all too likely to lose confidence in her own capacity to nourish the child and often suffers a spontaneous inhibition not only of her milk production but of the flow itself. Many women stopped breast-feeding not just because they were discouraged from doing so by their doctors, but because they 'didn't have enough milk'. Their baby's first cries confirmed what they had already been led to believe: 'I can't satisfy him'.

If the arrival of bottle-feeding tended to deprive mothers of responsibility for the nourishment of their babies, it could also serve as a means of releasing them from the burden of feeding altogether. Just as in earlier days the wealthy had employed wet-nurses to suckle their babies for them, so now any baby could equally well be given his bottle by father, sister, or next-door neighbour. Bottle-feeding offered women freedom from the unpaid and undervalued work of child care, and the opportunity to seek paid work outside the home that would give them a sense of their own worth.

Sheila Kitzinger suggests that some women 'may prefer to feed artificially because the symbolic value of being able to use bottles and artificial formula is great for them'. Manufacturers of infant formula feeds, and notoriously the major manufacturers, seek to expand the overseas market for their products by exploiting the value of bottle-feeding as a status symbol, with catastrophic results in many Third World countries.

By giving free samples of babymilk to hospitals, the companies gain entry into a highly lucrative market. Once bottle-feeding starts, breast milk begins to dry up, and by the time the mother and baby leave hospital they are physically 'hooked'.

In countries where mothers have neither the money nor the hygienic conditions to carry out bottle-feeding satisfactorily, the addiction has savage consequences: severe malnutrition, diarrhoea, gastroenteritis and ultimately death. The tragedy is that the situation is entirely preventable, because breast-feeding is safe, free, and best for baby.*

Medical opinion on breast-feeding has now come full circle, of course, and such aggressive marketing techniques are no longer permitted in the UK. The advertising of formula feeds for the home market now tends to forestall criticism by admitting openly that 'breast is best', playing instead on the modern

---

* *New Internationalist*, October 1988, p. 26.

woman's right to 'freedom of choice'. What the advertisements never explain, of course, is that having once begun to use the bottle, there is no freedom of choice at all. Once bottle-feeding has been started, Western mothers and their babies are as surely hooked as their Third World counterparts.

Breast milk contains just the right mixture of proteins, minerals and vitamins for your baby, as well as antibodies against many infections. The milk is more easily digestible than any of the cow's milk preparations, and a breast-fed baby is therefore less prone to gastric upsets and less likely to be constipated. Breast milk is free, does not have to be sterilized, and is constantly on tap at precisely the right temperature, which means that your baby's first pangs of hunger can be satisfied without his having to wait for a bottle to be made up or warmed. There is evidence that breast-fed babies are less likely to suffer from allergies such as eczema and asthma.[*] Breast-feeding stimulates uterine contractions, assisting the stretched womb to reduce to its normal size and helping the mother to regain her former shape. Lastly, breast-feeding offers you and your baby the opportunity to enter into an intimate and mutually satisfying relationship.

It is very rare indeed that a breast-feeding mother does not have enough milk, and with the assistance of a good midwife or of a woman who has herself breast-fed to help through the first difficult days, few mothers experience any lasting difficulty with breast-feeding. Incorrect positioning of the baby at the breast (see page 68) is a common cause of problems: the baby does not get a good flow of milk and becomes hungry and frustrated, and his sucking makes the nipples sore but fails to stimulate milk production. Giving the baby supplementary feeds can also inhibit milk production. If you plan to have your baby in hospital it is very important that the staff know of your wish to breast-feed and that no additional drinks of any kind, not even water, are given. Extreme anxiety about the quantity or the quality of your milk supply can itself restrict your milk production. If this happens, it is important to examine your fears, share them with your partner, and ask for help from your

---

[*] Sheila Kitzinger, *The Experience of Breast Feeding* (1979), p. 29.

midwife or from a National Childbirth Trust counsellor (see below).

In exceptional cases, it may be impossible or undesirable to breast-feed, for medical reasons. Occasionally breast-feeding may have to be abandoned due to paediatric complications, such as harelip or cleft palate. Mothers are sometimes frightened or embarrassed by breast-feeding. And sometimes a mother makes the clear choice not to breast-feed, as is of course her right. Excellent counselling and advice on all aspects of breast-feeding, are available free of charge from the National Childbirth Trust. For information about your nearest counsellor, contact NCT, 9 Queensborough Terrace, London W2 3TB (tel: 01-221 3833).

Mothers who are unable to breast-feed may feel dismay that they cannot give their baby the best. But more important even than the antibodies and the vitamin content of breast milk is the spirit in which it is offered. A loving mother, tenderly cradling her newborn infant in her arms, and deriving satisfaction herself from feeding him, will be giving him the nourishment he needs whether she gives him breast or bottle.

Nutritional Value of Breast Milk

There is no doubt that even a few weeks of breast-feeding are very valuable for any baby. The first milk, called colostrum, has a special role to play in the health of the newborn child. It is produced during pregnancy, ready for the moment of birth. In the later stages of pregnancy you may find that a small amount of the thick, creamy (sometimes quite yellow) colostrum leaks from your breasts. Rich in valuable proteins and fats, colostrum also contains antibodies which will protect your baby from many viral, bacterial and respiratory infections, and will pass on your own immunity to many illnesses as long as you are fully breast-feeding.

Between three and five days after the birth, transitional milk, less creamy but still full of proteins and antibodies, is produced. By ten days your mature milk will have established itself. The appearance of this milk contributes to the fear some women have that their milk is not adequately nourishing their child. But its thin, watery, bluish look is exactly as it should be. Provided you have a healthy diet, your milk will be rich in amino-acids (proteins), enzymes, hormones, vitamins, iron, calcium, and many trace elements.

It is natural for most babies to lose some 10 per cent of their birth weight in the first week of life, but this is normally regained by about two weeks after birth. If your baby is content, produces six to eight wet nappies a day and looks to be thriving, you can be sure he is getting what he needs. He will have no need for anything extra, not even water. All his requirements are being met by your milk.

Unlike the uniform flow of milk from a bottle, the rate of the flow of milk from the breast slows markedly towards the end of a feed, giving the baby's delicate stomach an opportunity to process the large quantity of milk he has already swallowed. This slowing of the flow reduces the likelihood of colic* (see page 77), and also explains why breast-fed babies rarely need to be winded, whereas bottle-fed babies must be winded carefully after every feed, and often 'posset' or bring up a proportion of the feed as curds.

Psychological Benefits of Breast-feeding

What psychologists call 'bonding' is the formation of a primal attachment to the mother which will serve as a prototype of relationship for the rest of a baby's life. Just as your baby is born into the world without a fully developed ability to fight harmful micro-organisms on his own, so too he has an undeveloped capacity to tolerate stimulation. Bright lights, harsh sounds, cold air, lack of bodily support, can all catapult him into a state of great anxiety. He needs to be enveloped gently by your body to ease his transition from an environment in which he was completely protected and his every need spontaneously met, to one in which he can feel extremely exposed.

If instead of being left to struggle on his own he is quietly

---

* Sheila Kitzinger, *The Experience of Breast Feeding*, p. 22.

allowed to rediscover your body, he will find a place that he knows is safe. As soon as he is born he will instinctively begin to 'root', and will find your nipple in his own time. This is a process in which he actively participates. Lactation is spontaneous, but breast-feeding requires relationship.

It is a mutually satisfying activity. Your breasts fill up and you long to have them emptied. Your baby's stomach empties and he longs to have it filled. You both give and you both receive. The gratification of his longing and the satisfaction of his hunger make your baby feel that all is well with the world. Feeding is his first experience, and the manner in which he is fed will have a profound bearing on how he perceives his world; on whether he senses a persecutory, hostile environment or a loving, caring one.

Breast-feeding is an intimate act in which each partner responds to the subtly changing needs of the other. It is this sexual aspect of breast-feeding with which some women find difficulty, but if it can be enjoyed, not as a substitute for adult sexuality, but as an exhilarating exploration of what this new relationship has to offer, then both you and your baby will benefit. You will gain greater insight into your child's needs and he will learn the valuable lesson of forming a close, tender human relationship; he will be learning to love.

The capacity to form an attachment between you and your baby at this stage of his life lays the foundation for the capacity to separate satisfactorily later. The more fully your baby is allowed to be dependent on you now for the satisfaction of his needs, the more easily will he later achieve independence, from the basis of a fundamental sense of security and trust in the world. And the more closely attuned you are to your baby's ever-changing needs, the better able you will be to recognize when he is ready to be more independent.

These feelings can be nurtured in bottle-fed babies too, but it is more difficult. Unless a bottle-fed baby is sometimes held closely against his mother's naked bosom, he will be unable to read the emotional messages which are subtly transmitted through his mother's musculature and sweat-glands. So if you are feeding your baby by bottle, try to do so consciously, actively, and tenderly. Do not simply allow the bottle to do the feeding.

How Often to Feed

It is the instinctive rooting and sucking of a baby in the hours immediately after his birth that activate the hormones which regulate the production and flow of milk. If you begin feeding as soon after birth as your baby is ready, you will also establish a rapport between you while your breasts are still soft and it is therefore easier to position your baby correctly.

Feed your baby whenever he wants to be fed; otherwise you are likely to find you have a diminishing milk supply and a dissatisfied, fretful baby who is not thriving. Nature has provided us with a beautifully balanced system of supply and demand. The more your baby sucks the more milk you will produce, so if you put him to feed whenever he is hungry, and let him feed for as long as he wants, he will be satisfied. There are often 'growing spurts' at around 5 days, 6 weeks, 3 months and 6 months, when there is an increased demand for milk. This is a time to settle down with your baby, putting aside for a few days as many other activities as you can, and feed as much as he wants. Very soon your supply of milk will increase to meet your baby's increased requirements, and he should be able to get what he needs in a series of clearly defined 'feeds' again.

Your baby needs to suck not only for nourishment but also for comfort. He is able to arrest the flow of milk when he does not need to feed, but needs to be close to you. And it is important to remember that every baby is unique: one will suck for hours drawing the same quantity of milk that another will take in twenty minutes. To put your baby at each breast for a predetermined length of time will interfere with the establishment of his feeding rhythm. Because the composition of breast milk at the beginning of a feed is different from that of milk at the end of a feed, it is best to let your baby suck as much as he wants from one breast before offering him the other. It may be that he only takes one breast at a particular feed. Do not worry; just remember to begin the next feed from the other side.

Every baby is different, and each one needs to feed or to be comforted in a different way. Some babies will happily wait three or four hours between feeds, while others will want to feed constantly. You will come to understand your own baby's rhythms intimately. When he is secure in the knowledge that his needs are taken seriously he will be able to tolerate the frustration of having to wait a bit for his feed, and you can begin to allow your own needs to surface. Rather than insisting that he feed strictly to a routine, or conversely becoming slave to his demands, feeding becomes a negotiation, in which you both learn to respect and respond to each other's changing needs.

Night feeds must also be negotiated between you. Some babies feed every hour for many months and some sleep through the night from the beginning. You will eventually convey to your child your own need to sleep, and together you will arrive at an arrangement which balances your separate needs.

Problems with Breast-feeding

Breast milk is produced in special glandular cells grouped in bundles in your breasts. It is passed from these cells along a network of tubes, called ducts, to the nipples. When your milk first 'comes in', your breasts may become engorged; hard and sore, and so swollen that the nipples virtually disappear. This is a result of the sudden increase in the flow of blood to the breasts, required for the production of the milk. It is perhaps the most difficult phase of breast-feeding, when some mothers give up, and many more think of doing so. It can be very painful; if a baby is unable to 'latch on' to swollen breasts he will probably be crying; and you are very likely to be tearful yourself as a result of hormonal changes brought about by lactation, and in a natural response to the release of tension after the strains of labour. If you persevere, these miserable moments will be well behind you after a couple of weeks.

'Latching on' is a term used to describe the correct meeting of mouth and breast, which is essential for the successful establishment of breast-feeding. Make sure that your baby has all of the nipple and most of the lower part of the areola (the dark area around the nipple) in his mouth, or his sucking will make you very sore. When your baby is properly latched on, you will see the tip of his ear wiggle as he sucks. If only his cheeks are moving in and out, he is probably not 'on' correctly. Your midwife will be able to help you with different positions. However, if you are engorged, it will be necessary to relieve your breasts of their intense discomfort and tightness before your baby can feed.

One way of relieving engorgement is to apply hot flannels to your breasts or to soak in a hot bath to get the milk flowing and relieve some of the pressure. Another way is by expressing a bit of the milk. This can be done by stroking firmly from a couple of inches above the nipple down to the areola, then pushing in and up to release the milk, while supporting the breast from below. Occasionally one of the milk ducts gets blocked, causing the milk to pool above it and creating a hard, tender lump in your breast. Massaging with a gentle circular motion from above the lump down towards your nipple will help get the blood flowing and relax the surrounding tissue, so dissipating the lump. If this persists and you become feverish, or feel as if you are getting the flu, an infection may be developing and you should contact your midwife or doctor straight away.

The problem of sore nipples is very common when breast-feeding is first being established. You will need to wear a good supporting bra when your milk comes in, but it is also important to air your nipples as much as possible to keep them dry. If they are allowed to remain for long periods in a damp bra they will certainly become sore. Calendula tincture, available from most health food shops, diluted in boiled water and dabbed on with cotton wool, can be very soothing. It is better not to use soap on your nipples as this dries up your body's natural oils. If you do wash your breasts with soap, rub a little almond oil into your nipples afterwards. Continue to feed, because your baby's saliva is very healing.

If you feel a sudden sharp pain in your nipple when your baby latches on, you probably have a crack. This can be very painful indeed. Calendula tincture and vitamin E oil both help with healing. If a crack is deep, contact your midwife or doctor. You may need to feed from the other side temporarily, and express milk from the sore breast. Some women find nipple shields (little latex covers worn over the ends of the breasts) helpful as a temporary measure until the crack heals. They should not be worn for long periods of time as a baby does not get the same amount of milk from a feed when they are worn. You will also need to wash and sterilize them after use.

Whatever problems you may be having in establishing breast-feeding, resist the temptation to supplement your own milk with formula milk or with other drinks of any kind, as this will only 'confuse' your breasts into 'thinking' that your baby's demand for milk is decreasing, and they will produce correspondingly less milk.

Each time your baby comes to your breast for a feed and the milk begins to flow, you will feel a tingling or tight feeling in your breasts. What you are feeling is the contraction of the milk glands, forcing the milk into the ducts. In some women the other breast than that from which the baby is sucking flows as well. And sometimes this 'let-down' reflex is stimulated by your baby's (or even another baby's) cries.

In order for your milk to flow you must be relaxed; if you are feeling at all tense about breast-feeding, practise the breathing and relaxation techniques you learned for labour. When you sit to feed, make sure you are in a position where you will be comfortable for some time, with your back well supported and your legs raised on a cushion or stool. You may need to raise your baby to your breast with the help of a cushion rather than bending to him, or you may find it more comfortable when both you and your baby lie down facing one another. Anxiety or embarrassment about feeding in front of others will also inhibit the flow of your milk. The company and support of other breast-feeding mothers can be helpful with this, but in the meantime make sure that you can feed in a relaxed way, and if necessary take your baby to a quiet place. Together you will build your confidence and come to experience the joy that feeding brings when it flows smoothly.

Food and Drink for Breast-feeding

It is certainly possible for a mother to breast-feed adequately without being on a special diet herself, as mothers around the world have always done, with diverse dietary habits, lifestyles, appetites and ranges of available food. However, if you try to get your figure back to normal while breast-feeding, rather than continuing to eat nutritiously, not only will you produce less milk, but you will become depleted, and eventually exhausted and depressed. As in pregnancy, whatever your baby requires to make him grow strong and healthy will pass to him from your reserves; if you do not have enough for the two of you, you will be the one to suffer. You are still 'eating for two' as you were when you were pregnant, but now in terms of actual quantity too: your baby's requirements for about 600 calories a day will be supplied by your milk and you will need that many extra calories yourself.

You may already be exhausted from the sleeplessness of the latter stages of pregnancy and from the enormous physical and emotional stresses of labour. The first weeks of adjusting to the presence of a new baby is a time to attend particularly closely to your own diet, in order to establish the high levels of energy you will need over the coming months and years. Do not jeopardize your health by ignoring your bodily needs now, simply because you 'don't have the time'.

You will certainly be busy, but you can still eat well. Try to have one good hot meal each day, which in the first weeks you will need to have cooked for you, by partner, family, or friend. Follow the guidelines given in Chapter 1, and ensure – particularly at this time – that the basis of your diet is a good varied supply of unrefined carbohydrates. It is the carbohydrates in your food which will supply the calories you need, both for your own energy and to produce plentiful milk for your baby. Be careful to preserve the quality of protein in your diet too, especially if you are not eating meat or dairy products; protein is also necessary for the production of healthy milk, and will speed your healing from labour.

One good meal a day is essential, but eat as much as you feel like through the day as well. Your snacks will need to be simple but should also be wholesome and nutritious. Baked potatoes, wholemeal bread or toast, cheese, nuts, raw fruit and vegetables; these and many other simple foods make good easy snacks. Include foods rich in vitamin C, such as citrus fruits, potatoes and fresh green vegetables, as this is the only vitamin passed directly through your milk to your baby. If you do not take in any vitamin C during the day, neither will he, and he needs plenty to help him resist infection and grow healthy tissues, and to aid his absorption of iron.

Eating little and often continues to be important when breast-feeding, particularly if you are feeling tired or depressed: it maintains your blood sugar level and increases your milk supply. You may have six small meals a day, or three regular meals, with snacks in between. After a feed, you may find that you are ravenous. Rather than eating chocolate or biscuits, which may give you a temporary boost but will leave you further run down, have a sandwich of wholemeal bread spread with peanut butter, or an apple and a piece of cheese. Keep a bowl of fresh fruit (already washed) or of dried fruit and nuts by your side when you feed to provide an easy way to nibble when you become hungry.

You will, for the first three or four months at least, need to be available for your baby whenever he calls, and this will make the preparation of elaborate meals difficult. A one-pot stew or soup is far less fuss than a variety of separate dishes. Roughly chopped raw vegetables are easier to prepare than a complicated salad. This is especially a time to involve your partner in the sharing of food preparation. And when friends and relations come to visit do not hesitate to ask them to prepare a meal, leaving you the time to be with your baby. Certainly avoid tiring yourself out by making extra food and drinks for the visitors who come to admire your new baby.

You may find that you need to drink more than usual during the months of breast-feeding, and especially while actually feeding you may become very thirsty. Make sure you have a drink by your side *before* you start to feed, or you are likely to find yourself longing for your baby to finish so that you can have a drink yourself. Rather than drinking coffee, tea or Coca-cola, all of which contain caffeine and will make your baby restless and sleepless, drink plenty of unsweetened fruit juices and herbal teas. There is a wide selection of concentrated fruit juices on the market that only need the addition of spring water or filtered water to make a delicious drink, hot or cold. Camomile tea relaxes both body and mind, and is therefore a good companion throughout breast-feeding.

Medicines, laxatives, alcohol and nicotine will all pass through the milk to your baby. Never take any medicine without first checking with your midwife or doctor. If you were a heavy smoker, you may have stopped or at least cut down the number of cigarettes you smoked during pregnancy, and it will be wise to continue with this for as long as you breast-feed, as your nicotine dependency can become your baby's. The occasional glass of wine probably does no harm, indeed there is iron in red wine. And a glass of stout, rich in B vitamins, has long been recommended for an increased supply of breast milk.

With the exceptions that we have mentioned, there is really nothing you should not eat when breast-feeding. You will probably receive all kinds of advice about onions and garlic, and spicy foods, but you can in fact follow your own tastes and appetite, and it is really only necessary to remember to eat nothing in excess. If you eat a new food, particularly one that you did not eat in pregnancy, watch carefully for any effect it may have on your baby. If a particular food upsets him he may be more restless than usual, may have a stomach upset in which he produces frothy green stools, or he may develop a rash. Eliminate the particular food you suspect and notice if this makes a difference.

Although the causes of colic are not fully understood, some breast-fed babies do get over colic if their mothers give up cow's milk and cow's milk products. The large protein molecules of cow's milk, ideally suited to the rearing of young calves, are less than ideal for human babies. This is the cause of the difficulties many babies experience with cow's milk formula feeds, but it appears that some breast-fed babies suffer similar reactions to the small quantities of the larger proteins which pass through their mothers' milk. Sheep and goat's milk contain a smaller protein more easily absorbed by a baby's stomach, and as well as goat's milk itself (often frozen), many delicious sheep and goat's cheeses and yoghurts are now widely available. It is certainly not true that breast-feeding mothers need to drink milk to make milk, but milk is a valuable source of protein, and if you cut out dairy products altogether you must be sure to get sufficient protein either from meat or from the correct combination of whole grains, pulses, seeds and nuts (see page 42).

A history of allergies in either of the parent's backgrounds is another very good reason for the mother to eliminate all cow's milk and its products from her diet for the duration of breast-feeding. Food allergies, the most common of which are to cow's milk, eggs, wheat and citrus fruits, are often the first irritants in the development of more general allergic problems. As long as you are solely breast-feeding, you can regulate what your baby takes in by careful attention to your own diet. When moving on to mixed feeding you will have to introduce foods carefully, one at a time (see Chapter 4). If you are already bottle-feeding and discover that your baby is allergic to cow's milk, there are several excellent soya-based formula feeds on the market, although some babies are unfortunately allergic to these too. If there is a history of allergies in the family, it is much better to breast-feed if you possibly can.

You cannot care thoroughly for your baby if your own needs are ignored. To nourish yourself properly while you breast-feed shows your baby that you care for your body and its needs, and teaches him that your own welfare is a necessary part of your care for him. Breast milk is the best food a baby can have, provided it is given by a mother who herself has the reserves of physical and emotional strength to feed with love. A poorly nourished mother nourishes her baby at her own expense; an activity which should be a source of rich contentment to both her and her child will distress and weaken her, and bring resentment between them.

Expressing Breast Milk

Some couples choose to share, at least in part, the pleasures and the strain of feeding. If this is to be done with a breast-fed child, then milk will have to be expressed so that the partner can give the feed from a bottle. A mother who regularly has to be away from her baby but who does not want to stop breast-feeding will also need to express milk, not just to provide the feed for which she will be absent, but also to keep up her supply of milk: if a formula feed is given while she is away her breasts will 'think' the baby's demand has dropped and she will soon find her supply of milk decreasing. Even if you can be with your baby all the time, it is good to have an alternative way of giving him your breast milk should you ever want or need to leave him for a few hours.

Small amounts of milk can be expressed by hand (see page 69), but many women find this method suitable only for relieving engorged breasts. For the regular collection of amounts suitable for a full feed, a hand or electric pump may be used. There are many types of hand pumps on the market. A simple one is operated by rhythmically squeezing a rubber balloon, which mimics the baby's sucking and deposits the milk in a wide-necked feeding bottle.

Breast milk can be stored in the refrigerator for twenty-four hours. One make of pump comes complete with freezer bags just the right shape and size for a small bottle. If you do intend to freeze breast milk and have only an ordinary refrigerator with a small freezing compartment, do not keep the milk for more than one week, as it could become sour. Electric pumps can be rented from the National Childbirth Trust (see page 64).

Attention to hygiene is very important whenever milk is expressed. Milk as it comes straight from the breast is sterile, and even the natural oils on the nipple contain antibacterial agents. Once the milk is outside the breast, however, it becomes highly susceptible to invasion by micro-organisms that can give your baby gastro-enteritis (see page 82), so it is very important that any bottle or container into which the milk is expressed, and all parts of the pump itself, are carefully washed and sterilized. Expressed milk should never be left standing at room temperature, either before or after refrigeration or freezing.

It should be said that not all women find it easy or pleasant to express their breast milk. In contrast to the comfortable closeness and warmth of feeding itself, the use of a breast-pump can seem coldly functional, and the 'let-down' of milk may not be as easy as with an ordinary feed, making the sucking of the pump uncomfortable, and even painful. Some women happily express a whole feed every day, but try it out before committing yourself to plans which require you to express milk.

Bottle-feeding

Feeding is an important element of the bonding between mother and baby which is crucial to a baby's psychological well-being (see page 65). This is true whether a baby is breast- or bottle-fed. In fact, if you are bottle-feeding it is probably even more important to pay attention to the way in which you feed than if you are breast-feeding. The eyes of a new-born baby focus at twelve inches, just the distance required for him to see his mother's face clearly while suckling at her breast. Hold him against your breast to bottle-feed too. If he is fed propped up in his chair or on pillows, not only is there a greater risk of his choking, but he will miss out on this first vital stage in the formation of his early relationship with you, and with the world you represent to him. He will feel alone, and will begin to suffer all the anxieties associated with loneliness. Hold him closely and tenderly as you feed him.

Just as with breast-feeding, it may take some time for you to be able to relax while feeding your baby, and to enjoy your regular sessions together. But the pleasure you take in feeding him is an important part of the growing relationship between you, and you should give yourself time for this satisfaction to develop. Always try to settle down in a comfortable position, and do not limit the length of the feed to the time it takes your baby to swallow a bottle-full of milk.

Bottle-feeding does enable a partner or a friend to share the strain as well as the enjoyment of feeding and holding a warm and contented baby. However, too many attendants bewilder and upset babies, who have a limited capacity for attachment. Always remember that your baby needs to form one strong, primary feeding relationship.

For babies who are to be bottle-fed, whether from choice or necessity, there are a number of baby milks on the market. These are modified cow's milk formulations, designed to be chemically as close as possible to human milk. One of these formula feeds, carefully chosen in consultation with your health visitor, will provide all the nutrients your baby will need until he is ready for solid foods. It is essential that an infant formula is *always* used, rather than either a 'follow-on' formula, ordinary cow's milk, or ordinary soya milk, all of which are perfectly suitable as supplements to a full solid diet, but which are unable on their own to meet all the nutritional requirements of a growing baby. Many mothers choose to supplement solids for the whole of the first year with the same formula milk they used for bottle-feeding.

If a bottle-fed baby does not thrive, vomits after each feed, has diarrhoea, or develops skin rashes, this may be caused by an allergy to the cow's milk of his formula (see page 73), and you will need to try one of the soya-based formula milks (not to be confused with ordinary soya milk in cartons) which can be bought in most chemists, but which are also available on prescription. Some brands of cow's milk formula are usually stocked by baby clinics, where they can be bought in bulk at a discount. It is unwise to switch to a different formula unless there is a very good reason, as switching may in itself upset your baby's sensitive digestion.

'Three-month colic', as it is commonly called, is characterized by frequent discomfort or pain after feeds. A colicky baby will turn beet-red and scream, drawing his knees to his chest and writhing in pain within minutes of feeding. This often happens at about the same time each day, commonly in the early evening, leaving parents drained, exhausted, and sometimes quite desperate. Although breast-fed babies may suffer in this way (see page 73), the incidence of colic among bottle-fed babies is very much higher. If your baby develops colic, ask your doctor to give you a prescription for a soya-based formula feed, and make sure that he gets no cow's milk products at all. Avoid the 'traditional' remedy of Gripe Water, which relies on a powerful dose of alcohol to dull the baby's pain.

There has been concern recently about the levels of aluminium found in some formula feeds. Aluminium does not act as an acute poison, but there is now considerable evidence that it accelerates the ageing process, weakening the bones by displacing calcium, and increasing the risk of brain disorders such as Alzheimer's disease. Poorly functioning kidneys (including the immature kidneys of premature and very young babies) can allow the metal to build up in the body. Levels of aluminium are highest in the soya-based formula feeds, although all brands are implicated, as are other baby foods. Other sources are tap water, unlacquered aluminium cans, and aluminium pans and kettles, which should not be used for your baby's drinks or meals at all.

How Much Formula Milk to Give

Some mothers actually choose to bottle-feed as a way of relieving their anxiety about how much milk their babies are drinking, gaining reassurance from seeing the clearly marked ounces draining from the bottle. However, babies' needs vary so widely that it is impossible to say how much milk any individual baby should have. The manufacturers of formula feeds normally recommend giving 2½–3 fluid ounces per pound of body weight in each 24-hour period. There is no harm in having this as a rough guide, but if you impose a predetermined number of ounces of feed on your baby you are likely to find either that he is often disgruntled and dissatisfied because he has not had as much as he would have liked, or that he is getting fat because he is always given more than he really requires. In either case, he will be deprived of the satisfaction and reassurance of a flexible and constantly evolving feeding pattern based on his individual digestive needs. Feed a bottle-fed baby in the same way you would a breast-fed baby: on demand, whenever he asks for it, and only as much as he wants. He will not take more than he needs, and will stop when he has had enough. There is no need to slap his feet or tickle his chin as he falls asleep on the bottle, to get him to 'finish' a feed.

Until the moment of birth your baby was fed automatically, his stomach continuously topped up. Now he has to get used to a new pattern of feeding, as his stomach slowly empties between feeds, and is then filled. It will take 3–4 weeks for your baby's own digestive rhythm to emerge, and for you to know when he requires full feeds and when he needs less. If you worry about 'giving in' to your baby's demands and try to impose control over his feeding by forcing him to adhere to a fixed routine, you are much more likely to end up with a demanding baby than if you feed on demand. A baby who is fed on demand knows his own requirements and learns to express them in the confidence that they will be satisfied.

Bottle-feeding Equipment and Routine

How much equipment you buy depends on how you plan to organize the sterilization of bottles and equipment. Specially made sterilizing units are available, but tend to be expensive, and it is possible to manage perfectly well with the simpler equipment listed here:

2 straight-edged plastic knives

Bottle-cleaning brush

8–10 plastic bottles with teat-covers. Measurements should be clearly marked on the side of the bottles

Tray to keep equipment organized

2 large plastic containers with tight-fitting lids for sterilizing. These should be large enough to hold half your equipment totally submerged in sterilant

10 teats of clear silicone rather than of latex. Silicone is longer-lasting and more hygienic; it does not crack, blister or discolour. Teats are available with a valve which allows air to enter the bottle as the baby sucks, to prevent a vacuum forming

Sterilizing tablets, solution, or crystals, available from chemists.

The advantage of using two sterilizing containers is that it enables you to organize sterilizing twice daily, which means that you will always have enough clean and sterile bottles and teats ready for use. Wash and sterilize night-time bottles in the mornings, and day-time bottles in the evenings, and you should never need to use a bottle which has been immersed in sterilant for less than the required length of time (see page 82 for more detailed discussion of washing and sterilizing procedures).

The correct measurement of water and formula powder is extremely important when bottles are being given as a baby's sole food. The milk should be made up precisely as intended, using only the measuring scoop provided and carefully following the directions on the tin. Never mix a feed with anything other than cooled boiled water, and never attempt to 'enrich' it by adding an extra scoop of powder, or by packing or heaping the scoop. You may have been told that an 'extra rich' feed will make your baby sleep longer, but it will give him too much salt for the volume of liquid consumed, and too many calories, and can lead to kidney and even brain damage. Similarly, a watered-down feed will leave your baby dissatisfied and undernourished. Never heat up a cold bottle of milk by adding boiling water to it, as this will cause a dangerous dilution of your baby's food.

Typically, a bottle-feed is made up following these steps:

- Boil water and let it cool to slightly over 'hand-hot'
- Wash hands thoroughly
- Remove bottle and teat from sterilizing container, and rinse with boiled water
- Using the graduated marks on the side of the bottle, fill it to the required level with cooled boiled water. Bring the bottle up to eye level to ensure correct measurement
- Measure the exact amount of milk powder using the scoop provided. Without packing down the powder, level off each scoopful with a straight-edged knife
- Add each scoop of powder one by one to the water in the bottle

■ Screw on the cap of the bottle tightly, and shake until all lumps have dispersed and dissolved.

Four or five bottles can be made up at one time and kept refrigerated until required. When needed, stand the bottle in a jug of hot (just boiled) water to warm. Shake the bottle to distribute the heat evenly, and sprinkle a few drops on the inside of your wrist. It should be just blood temperature, and should therefore feel neither warm nor cool on your skin. Do not keep the milk warm for more than half an hour before feeding it to your baby, and never put a bottle back in the refrigerator for later use once it has been warmed.

If you gently touch your baby's cheek with your finger or with the teat of the bottle he will instinctively root, as a breast-fed baby does for the nipple, and will turn towards you to be fed. Make sure that the teat is always full of milk. If a valveless teat is used, a vacuum will form in the bottle as the baby sucks, and eventually the teat will flatten, slowing or completely blocking the flow of milk, and frustrating your baby. Every minute or two you will have to remove the teat from his mouth completely to allow air to flow back into the bottle.

The size of the hole in the teat of his bottle should match the strength of your baby's sucking. Too large a hole can lead to indigestion, and may cause a very young baby to choke. If the hole is too small, your baby will not only be frustrated in his attempts to satisfy his hunger, but he is also likely to suck in air, giving himself wind. Teats are available with holes of three different sizes: small ('slow flow'), medium and large. The appropriate size of teat hole is generally proportional to the size of the baby: a small, poorly baby will need to start with the slowest flowing teat, and will progress to larger hole sizes as he grows; a big baby may need a medium-flow teat from soon after birth. If in doubt, it is best to buy teats with smaller holes; you can if necessary enlarge the hole in a teat by gently passing a red-hot needle through it.

Bottle-fed babies tend to need 'winding'. Wind your baby half-way through each feed and then again at the end of the feed, bringing him upright and holding him close to you, gently rubbing his back. It is not necessary to slap or even to pat him, in order to help him bring up wind.

Unlike breast-fed babies, bottle-fed babies do sometimes need drinks of cooled boiled water in addition to their formula feeds. Your baby may cry out of thirst as well as out of hunger. Never offer a drink of water in place of a feed, but rather between feeds, allowing him to drink as little or as much as he wants. As long as you are fully bottle-feeding, he will be getting all the nourishment he needs from his formula milk, so do not offer drinks other than water. It is only when you start to wean, when your baby is beginning to take solid foods, that you may wish to offer other drinks as a source of additional nourishment (see page 89).

Hygiene and Safety

Strict attention to cleanliness is as important when bottle-feeding as the correct dilution of the formula powder. Sweet, warm milk provides an ideal medium for bacteria to flourish. These micro-organisms multiply rapidly, and quantities that might pass unnoticed in an adult may overwhelm the partially developed immune and digestive systems of a young baby, leading to gastro-enteritis. A baby's stools are always variable, but if your baby has green, frothy diarrhoea, and if at the same time he seems ill, loses his appetite and perhaps vomits, these may be signs of gastro-enteritis and you should seek medical advice immediately. Meanwhile offer your baby as much cooled boiled water as he will drink, as babies suffering from gastro-enteritis dehydrate very quickly.

All bottles, teats, plastic knives, measuring jugs and scoops – anything which comes into contact with the milk powder or the made-up milk – must be thoroughly washed, and sterilized by total immersion either in a chemical sterilizing solution or in boiling water for at least twenty minutes. Make sure that teats, bottles and bottle brushes are all thoroughly cleaned each time they are used, and as soon after the feed as possible. Rinse the bottle and the teat in cold water, wash carefully with hot soapy water, using the bottle brush to reach corners and lips of the teat and around the threaded parts of bottle and cap. The teat should be turned inside out and scrubbed to remove the greasy film left by the milk. Then rinse both teat and bottle again to remove all soap, and completely immerse them in sterilizing solution, making sure that they contain no bubbles of air in which bacteria might breed. Teats should be held below the surface of the solution by the cap of the bottle, again making sure that this does not contain a pocket of air. Sterilant should be changed according to the manufacturer's instructions, normally every twenty-four hours.

Milk that remains in a bottle at the end of a feed should always be tipped away, and refrigerated bottles of milk made up in advance should never be kept longer than twenty-four hours. Make a habit of clearing out any milk left in the refrigerator at the same time each day, and emptying and washing the bottles.

As a baby gets older, it is easy to slip into the habit of allowing him to carry his bottle around with him, feeding himself, but there are important reasons for avoiding this practice. A bottle of formula feed will be particularly prone to bacterial infestation if it is carried around uncovered, set down when he needs both hands, and picked up again later. Formula milk also contains sugars, and if your baby is sucking at his bottle off and on all afternoon or evening his teeth are likely to decay. All in all, it is best to keep the association of his formula bottle feeds with you, and with the special feeding times you share with him.

Bacteria multiply far more rapidly in warm milk, so never warm up a bottle in advance, as you might perhaps be tempted to do for a night feed. Instead keep a bottle ready made up but refrigerated, and for speedy heating prepare a thermos flask of hot water. Microwave ovens provide another quick way of heating up refrigerated feeds but should not be used for heating milk. You should be *sure* to test the temperature of the milk on your wrist before giving it to your baby. The milk itself will be heated more rapidly than the bottle, and the temperature of the bottle could mislead you into feeding milk so hot that it would scald his mouth. Always shake the bottle before testing to distribute the heat evenly.

If your home is equipped with a water-softening system, use a low-sodium, low-mineral content bottled spring water for all your baby's drinks and feeds, unless you can arrange for one tap to give unsoftened *mains* water (not cold water from a storage tank), in which case you may use this. Chemical water softeners contain sodium which can cause dehydration, and eventually kidney damage, in young babies.

Although cleanliness and attention to hygiene of course remain important, sterilization is not normally necessary after six months if the baby is well and thriving, and mains water used for formula feeds or other drinks will no longer need to be boiled. For premature, poorly, or very small babies, it is better to continue sterilizing all equipment and boiling all water for the whole of the first year.

Feeding on the Move

Travelling presents no major difficulties to breast-feeding mothers and their babies, as soon after the birth as they feel ready to venture out. Long journeys are a problem, however, for bottle-fed babies for as long as all their bottles and feeding equipment need to be sterilized. Once that point is passed (see above), then still bottled spring water can be used to make up feeds, and they too can easily take to the open road!

Whether you are breast- or bottle-feeding, and whether on a short or a long journey, various tips are worth following. Be very careful about giving your baby milk either from breast or bottle while you are actually moving, as this is likely to make him sick. In a car, it is usually best to stop for a feed, and for a short time after the feed. If he needs a drink while you are driving, it is better to give plain water. Never try to keep bottles warm in an insulated bag. If you have such a bag, it is better to use it to keep a bottle or two *cold*, for warming later. If you are unable to warm it, it is still better for your child to drink a cold bottle than to have a bottle that has been kept warm for more than half an hour. Try to disrupt your baby's routine as little as possible. Arrange your stops to allow him to feed at his regular times, and make yourself and him as comfortable as you can for his feeds as you would at home, even though you may be in a very different situation.

If you are able to plan your stops in advance, look out for hotels, B-and-Bs, and restaurants which advertise themselves as being set up to cater for children. Motorway service station cafeterias are normally willing to heat bottles or jars of food. If all else fails, most hotel rooms are equipped with an electric kettle, and you can heat a bottle by standing it in the freshly boiled kettle *after* it has been switched off.

4 Transition to Solid Foods

When to Introduce Solid Foods

The gradual process of weaning takes many months to complete. It starts with the introduction of food and drinks other than milk and water, and ends when the baby is eating a fully established diet of varied solid foods and taking all her drinks, including milk, from a cup. To wean your baby is to accustom her to foods other than milk, and to the absence of sucking as a source of sustenance and comfort. As with other developmental processes, the transition to solid foods is likely to be made most smoothly when the child is allowed to set the pace of change. There is no special time to begin weaning; solids can be introduced whenever your baby is ready for them. But this is a major step for her which she will handle best in a safe and secure environment, so give her her first solids at home, and pick a time when she is neither unwell nor teething.

At some time between three and eight months the volume of milk required to satisfy your baby's growing nutritional needs will exceed the capacity of her stomach, and she will start to want a more concentrated food. Before three months, her digestive system will be unable to process anything other than milk, and solid foods will inhibit the absorption of the milk she needs. Premature introduction of solid foods also increases the risk of gasto-enteritis and of long-term allergies (see page 100). If, on the other hand, you give your child no solid foods until she is already dissatisfied with milk alone, her hunger and frustration will make it difficult for her to adjust to a new way of eating. Premature and low birth-weight babies will usually take rather longer to be ready for solids. In general, babies will be ready around the time they reach a weight of 7 kilos (15lbs).

If you include your baby in your family mealtimes, you will notice her beginning to take an interest in what you eat. You may have fed her at mealtimes for months, and she will have continued to suck, oblivious of your eating. But one day she will turn from the breast or bottle and with intense curiosity follow the passage of your hand from plate to mouth with her eyes. She may even reach out for a fork or spoon. She will lick her lips, shake or suck her fists, or wiggle her toes in excitement at the sight of food, as she begins to realize that you put solid food in your mouth just as she takes milk in hers. If she is grumbly and dissatisfied even after full feeds, or if, having been sleeping through the night, she starts waking every couple of hours again, these may also be signs that she is beginning to need something more than milk.

Her first taste of solid food will excite and startle your baby, for she will be entering a new and unfamiliar world of sensation. When you feel that she is ready, choose an occasion when you can both be relaxed. She may find it easier to tackle this new experience in the middle of the day rather than in the morning or evening when she is likely to need her established routine. But most importantly, choose a time when your own confidence and calm will communicate themselves to her, and take it very slowly.

First solids are only tastes. When a child starts to take her first thin, runny, 'solid' foods she will still be getting all the nourishment she needs from her mother's milk or from the bottle, and it will be some time before she starts to take less milk. As long as she is still breast- or bottle-feeding at least four times a day her tastes of solid foods are simply a supplementary 'treat', slowly interesting her in and accustoming her to this very different form of feeding. Her appetite for these solid foods can at this stage vary enormously from meal to meal and from day to day without in any way affecting her health.

You may continue full breast- or bottle-feeding for many months, but this will depend on your baby's need, and her enthusiasm, for solid foods. Do not try to rush her into giving up her liquid feeds. Follow her lead, and you will both be better able to enjoy her gradual exploration of this exciting new world of tastes and textures.

What to Start With

First solids are in fact only semi-solid. They should be loose in consistency, bland in taste (at least to an adult), and smooth in texture. Cereal flours or flakes make good first foods because they can meet all these requirements, and contain plenty of calories. Thin porridges made from rice flour, or from rice or millet flakes, are ideal.

Introduce one new food at a time. Cereal should only be given once a day. Other first foods can include mashed banana or avocado, stewed and puréed apple or pear, and potato, pumpkin, carrot, swede, cauliflower or parsnip, boiled and blended. All these foods can be mashed or blended with a small amount of expressed breast milk, soya milk, or formula milk added to achieve the right consistency. Serve them at room temperature or only slightly warmer. At this early stage it is best to avoid cow's milk and cow's milk products, wheat, pulses, eggs, meat and fish, citrus fruits, yeast extract, and salt and sugar in any form. And if there is any food your baby seems not to like, then avoid that too for a couple of weeks before trying it again. Keep things simple. A little mashed carrot will make a good meal for your baby, and if you are cooking carrots for your own meal then it will be simple for you to prepare, too. Just remember not to season the vegetable until you have taken out her portion.

If your child has accepted her first tastes of solid food at four months, then by seven months she will probably be eating three meals a day, and will be ready for a wider variety of foods. She can now try lentils, peas and beans, barley and oats, greens, satsumas and oranges, eggs, fish, cheese, pasta and bread. As before, introduce a single new food at a time, and withdraw any food which she does not seem to like, or which upsets her stomach or causes a rash.

During the first year of your baby's life, milk of one kind or another will form an essential part of her diet, so always offer a drink of milk with or after every meal, either from the breast, from a bottle, or from a beaker or cup when she is ready for this. If she refuses milk except from the breast or bottle, you can use it to thin her food, or to make custards and puddings.

As she begins to eat more solids, moving on to three meals a day and drinking less milk, her need for other liquids to replace the water content of the milk will increase, particularly in warm weather. Plenty of liquids will give your baby's kidneys a good cleansing and prevent constipation, which is a common problem when starting solids. Do not assume that your child won't drink plain water. Good clean water (preferably filtered mains water or still spring water), at room temperature or slightly warmed, is quite acceptable to many children, and is certainly better for them than sweet drinks.

Some juices (such as apple and pear) are available as concentrates, and represent good value. All fruit and vegetable juices, whether concentrated or not, must be diluted for children. Bottled or freshly squeezed apple or carrot juice, for example, should be diluted with 10 parts water to 1 part of juice for six-month-olds, and may gradually be given at lower dilutions to about 5 parts water to 1 part juice from one year onwards. Concentrates should clearly be diluted even further; ½ a teaspoon of concentrated fruit juice is about right for a full 5 fl oz (¼ pint) beaker or bottle. Acidic juices such as orange and blackcurrant should not be used before the child is a year old, and should be introduced with caution then, as they sometimes provoke a rash or a stomach upset. Cooled and well-diluted herbal teas make good accompaniments to meals, or serve for a between-meals drink. Rosehip tea contains vitamin C. Camomile tea can be used to help settle teething pain, and is also a good drink to give at night-time awakenings for its calming effects.

There is certainly a place for the occasional use of manufactured baby foods. Many are perfectly wholesome, and the keeping qualities of meals in jars and tins (until opened) and the speed with which they can be heated make them useful in emergencies. The fact that sealed jars and tins do not need to be refrigerated also makes them ideal for picnics and journeys. Read the labels of these foods carefully. Do not be content to accept the 'no artificial colourings' flag on the label as evidence that the jar contains a healthy food for your child, but check the full list of ingredients. We suggest that you buy only meals in which *all* the ingredients are themselves foods which you recognize and would use at home yourself.

Since ready-made baby foods nowadays contain no chemical preservatives, extreme care must be taken over their storage once they have been opened – even those that come in re-sealable jars. If a meal has been heated in the jar or the tin, or if a baby has been fed directly from the jar, do not save the uneaten portion of the meal. If half the contents are removed from the jar when it is opened to be heated or to be fed from a bowl as it is, then if the container can be re-sealed the remainder may be stored in a refrigerator for up to twenty-four hours. This does *not* apply to meals which contain meat, which should be thrown out immediately if not eaten soon after opening.

Basic Methods: Cereals and Purées

Baby rice can be made from rice flour (whole ground rice), rice flakes, or from whole grain rice. The correct consistency for a tiny baby can be achieved directly by using rice flour, but if either flakes or whole grains are used the cooked cereal must be liquidized to achieve a thin, smooth porridge.

Using brown rice flour, which can be bought in most wholefood shops, could hardly be easier. Put 1 volume of the flour in a pan with 6 volumes of cold, unsweetened soya milk. The measure you use will depend on how much cereal you wish to make, but to begin with a level dessertspoon will give enough for you to freeze several portions in addition to what will be used immediately. Whisk flour and milk together with a fork, then bring slowly to the boil, stirring all the time. Remove the pan from the heat, cover it with a lid, and leave to stand for five minutes before serving.

A basic method for making porridge from any cereal flakes is given in Chapter 5 (see page 128). Use this method to make baby rice using rice flakes, adding a little extra liquid when the porridge is blended. If whole rice is to be used, simmer 2 oz (50g) of washed organic brown rice in 10 fl oz (275ml) of water in a covered pan for 1 hour, then liquidize the rice and remaining cooking water in a blender, adding a little breast, soya, or formula milk to achieve a suitable consistency. A similar thin porridge can be made from millet, millet flour or millet flakes. And as time goes by you can begin to combine this simple baby cereal with small quantities of puréed fruit or vegetables.

Non-organic fruits and root vegetables, such as apples and pears, potatoes and carrots, should always be peeled. All vegetables and fruits should be carefully washed, then diced or roughly chopped before steaming in a small amount of water (see page 125) until tender but not soft. Blend together with any remaining cooking water to retain nutrients lost during cooking. Add a little soya milk or plain boiled water as necessary to thin the purée.

There is no need to vary the texture or consistency of your baby's meal during the early, 'pre-teeth' stages of mixed feeding, and highly flavoured foods should be avoided. The different tastes and colours of a variety of simple, unseasoned cereal and vegetable meals will be exciting enough to her: the strong orange of the pumpkin; the rich scarlet of the beet; the muted green of the avocado. After a few months, her food will not need to be so finely puréed, and you can begin to vary the texture of her meals as well.

Quantities

This transitional stage is often a time when parents are particularly worried about the quantities of food their child is eating. As long as she is still taking the breast or bottle four or five times a day you can be confident that she is getting enough, however little solid food she eats. But if your baby takes enthusiastically to solids, then after a few weeks you will probably be giving her two meals of solids a day, following each with a milk feed to complete the meal. In a few weeks more you can try adding a third solid meal, and if she regularly accepts this her consumption of milk will almost certainly begin to decline.

When she is down to two or three liquid feeds, it may be hard to believe that she can survive on the tiny amounts of solid food she seems to take. A poorly child, who is badly 'off her food' for more than two or three days at a time, is clearly a proper cause for serious concern. But in the normal course of events any reasonably contented child, offered a plentiful variety of wholesome foods, will eat what she needs, and her development of healthy eating patterns is more likely to be damaged by her parents' continual and undue anxiety about the amount she eats than it is by actual undereating.

The best evidence of your ability to feed your child adequately, and of her ability to eat well, will be her general health and contentment. After six months it is no longer strictly necessary to have her regularly weighed, but if you are still worried about whether she is eating enough it may alleviate your anxiety to do so, and to see her steady weight gain. Keep a careful record of everything she actually eats each day, and see for yourself how much her appetite has grown over a couple of months, however dramatically it may have fluctuated in that time.

Give solids only once a day to begin with, and in minute quantities. Your baby will not know what to do with a mouthful of food at first, and will not need it for nourishment at this stage. It is enough for her to taste it, so just give her the tip of a spoon dipped in the food until she asks for more. The following suggestions will give a rough idea of appropriate quantities. For the first two weeks, offer up to a teaspoonful of rice cereal once a day. For the next couple of weeks, one teaspoon of rice cereal at one meal and one teaspoon of a bland puréed fruit or vegetable at another. For the next two weeks after that, offer as much as two teaspoons of cereal at one meal, adding a little puréed fruit to vary the flavour from time to time, and the same amount of fruit or vegetable purée at another. These are tiny quantities, but your baby's digestive system is still very delicate and requires some time to get used to foods other than milk. However enthusiastic she may be, if you give her much more than this you will undoubtedly both regret it later.

Finger Foods

Between six and eighteen months, the balance gradually shifts from being fed to eating. The onset of teething varies tremendously from child to child, but most children will begin biting and chewing somewhere between six and eight months. If you have started your baby on solids a few months earlier, then this may indicate that she is ready for a shift from purées to mashed, minced or finely chopped foods of a rougher texture. At about the same time she will begin to enjoy finger foods. Pieces of toasted bread are a good alternative to the heavily sweetened rusks sold in the shops. Bananas, peeled and pitted grapes, pieces of ripe pear or tomato, segments of satsuma, cheese, and any steamed and diced vegetable all make good finger foods, and provide a variety of tastes, colours and textures.

Your child will still need to be spoon-fed most of the time, but her desire to control the way she eats will be stimulated by finger foods, and her interest in exercising choice about what she eats will grow too. Around the time when she begins to feed herself, you are likely to find that she becomes more choosy about her food. She will have tasted at family mealtimes a wide range of adult foods of various flavours and textures. It is not surprising that she begins to weary of her rather uniform baby foods. The answer is not to 'spice up' her existing food by adding sugar, salt, or other flavourings, but to begin using new fruits and vegetables in different combinations, and perhaps blended to a slightly rougher consistency. Her meals at this stage can begin more closely to resemble your own.

Until she has a full set of teeth, you will see that she can only 'mumble' between her gums solid foods such as bread and cheese, rather than chewing them as you would, and she still needs to have the bulk of her food blended, if no longer to an absolutely smooth purée. Finger foods extend her food experience and her eating skills, giving her greatly increased scope for the exercise of food choice, but on their own they are not able to meet her nutritional needs. For her to take in sufficient volumes of food to satisfy her hunger you should continue to blend or mash her main meals. This is also important as a means of enabling you to manage the *combination* of foods eaten together in each meal, which is a nutritionally significant factor, particularly in relation to protein (see page 42). The proportion of finger foods that she eats will certainly increase, but you should continue to make blended meals available at every mealtime, ensuring not only that they are of good nutritional quality but also that they are sufficiently varied in flavour and texture to interest her.

Never leave a child alone while she is eating, particularly at this finger food stage. She is still learning how to manipulate pieces of food with her lips and tongue as well as with her fingers. Until all her teeth have come through, there is always a risk that she may choke (see page 134).

Equipment

It is worth taking care over the selection of equipment. It is probably a good idea to buy basic equipment before the birth, when you have time to choose carefully, but if you do not already have children of your own, ask a friend who has young children to go with you. Friends and relations with grown children are likely to have discarded but still perfectly serviceable equipment which they may be prepared to lend or pass on.

Unless she can already sit up, your child will suck her first tastes of solid food from a spoon while cradled in your arms, just as she is for a feed of milk from breast or bottle. All you will need in the way of equipment at this stage is a blender, a plastic spatula, a stainless-steel pot with lid, and some little (10 fl oz/275ml) freezer containers. While she is taking only a teaspoonful or two of food at a meal, you can use an ice-cube tray with separate plastic containers for each cube to freeze her miniature portions, if you are able to find such a thing (most manufacturers seem to have phased these out). Freezing a batch of cereal in portions will save considerable time and waste, and will mean that you always have a meal quickly available. Portions can be kept in the freezing compartment of a domestic refrigerator for a week. Reheat frozen meals thoroughly and then cool before serving. A little mashed fruit or puréed fruit or vegetable can be added as the meal is reheated.

High-chair   As soon as your child is able to sit up she can begin to sit at the table in a high-chair at mealtimes. Choose a high-chair with a tray of about the same height as the table at which you eat. It should be stable, which means that its legs must be splayed so that they are about six inches *outside* the line of the chair's seat. The tray should have a rail round it to prevent bowls from sliding off, or, better still, a raised rim all round, which will also help the child in her first attempts to pick up finger foods. Restraining straps should never be tightly fitted, but are necessary to prevent her from throwing herself overboard while you are at the other end of the room. By about eighteen months she will be ready for a 'booster' seat, which can be strapped to an ordinary kitchen chair so that she can eat at the table like everyone else.

Bibs   Absorbent towelling bibs are useful when a child first starts to drink from a teacher-beaker. The spout of the beaker does not cut off the flow of liquid when she stops sucking, as her mother's nipple or the teat of a bottle did, and she must learn to control the flow by tipping the beaker. Until she acquires this knack a good deal of the liquid will probably come back out again, and towelling bibs help to avoid the necessity of a complete change of clothes after each meal. They are useful in the same way during bouts of teething, particularly with the first few teeth, when heavy dribbling can rapidly soak a baby's clothes from chin to waist. On the other hand, plastic bibs are preferable once the bulk of what the baby spills is solid or semi-solid rather than liquid. They can be wiped off after a meal and only need to be washed every few days, whereas a towelling bib will usually have to go in the wash after a single meal. Two plastic bibs should be plenty: choose ones long enough to cover the baby down to the waist, and preferably with a pouch or pocket at the bottom to catch at least some of what is dropped.

Spoons   Spoons, bowls and beakers that a child is to use herself should of course be unbreakable. First spoons should be small (about half the size of a regular teaspoon), fairly shallow, and smooth-edged. It is worth buying a set of six or twelve, as they will undoubtedly get lost and broken, and you will anyway need two or three in the course of a single meal, as they are thrown on to the floor. By nine to twelve months, your baby will probably want to take bigger mouthfuls than a small spoon can hold. The white plastic disposable spoons used in many cafés are perfectly adequate at this stage, although they do not last very long; they can have sharp edges if they snap, so you must not let your child chew on them. Metal spoons are best avoided until the first eight teeth have been cut. Unlike plastic, metal conducts heat, so be careful that the spoon is the same temperature as her food.

Bowls   Plastic bowls with rubber suction rings or feet are available, but most children do not take long to work out how to release the suction, so it is probably not worth paying extra for this refinement. As with other feeding equipment for children, the important points to look for are that there are no sharp edges, and that the bowl is easy to clean, without awkward corners or rims where food might lodge. One bowl will probably be enough as children are generally happy to have each course of their meals served in the same plate, but your child may like to have two bowls of different colours for variety.

Beakers   The best kind of teacher-beaker has a threaded top that screws on to the base so that it will not fly off even when the beaker is thrown to the floor, and an interchangeable screw-on lid for leak-free transport in pocket or bag. Choose one with two handles, or with no handles: your child will need to use two hands to lift the beaker anyway, and will find a single handle awkward. If she has used a bottle, she will already have learned how to tip it up to make the liquid flow to the teat; if not, she will have to learn this now. In other respects, the action of drinking from a teacher-beaker is closer to that of drinking from an open cup or mug. The liquid pours freely from the spout when the beaker is tipped, but should not spill completely as a cup would. If your child drinks formula milk from her beaker, be extremely careful when washing it; undissolved lumps of the powder can get trapped inside the end of the spout where they are difficult to dislodge, and if left will form a breeding-ground for bacteria.

Mealtimes

Allowing and encouraging your baby to experiment with her food will help her to establish lasting healthy eating patterns. A child who is simply propped up or strapped in, the food ladled mechanically into her mouth and every spill immediately mopped up, may feel that feeding is something rather unpleasant done *to* her. On the other hand, if she is given the opportunity to explore her food in her own way and in her own time, she is more likely to feel that meals are events in which she can actively engage and which she can enjoy.

Your child's high-chair gives her her own vantage-point from which to observe your family meals. If she is compelled to stay in her high-chair she will probably come to hate it, and will resist being put into it when her own meal is ready. On the other hand she may enjoy sitting there while everyone else eats, even if her meal is finished. She may like to play where she can keep an eye on what is going on, so provide her with plenty of things to play with, whether toys or unbreakable (and blunt) tableware. And increasingly as she gets older she will want to sample your food, and can be given pieces of suitable foods on her tray. Include her as much as you can, and as much as she wants, in your adult meals.

A child's first attempts to feed herself often have more to do with her wish to imitate the adults she sees around her than with a desire to gain control over what she eats. But by the time she is eating some solid food three times a day, this will have become an important part of her diet. She will have realized that these new, strangely coloured soups, custards and fruit purées, with their astonishing range of flavours, also please and satisfy her in a way which only your breast or the bottle you gave her used to do. And having recognized her food as such, she will begin to explore the new possibilities of exercising choice in relation to food: choice about which food; about when and how quickly she eats; and about how the food gets from the bowl to her mouth.

From the time you first try her on solids, always use two spoons, one for her and one for you. To begin with she will probably be quite happy simply to hold her spoon while you feed her with the other. There is no need to persuade her to use the spoon properly; she will not have the coordination to do so yet, and will learn in her own time. She may start by using her spoon to feed you as you feed her. This is a useful game, so do not discourage her: she will learn how to balance and guide the spoon; she will enjoy sharing her food with you; and she will see that you think her food is good (if it is really unpleasant, you should not be giving it to her anyway).

It is with finger foods that she will learn to feed herself. She may try scooping blended foods into her mouth with her hand, but will probably find this frustrating, and if foods that she can pick up are offered she is likely to prefer these to practise her new skill. Once she has mastered the technique of picking up pieces of food and putting them in her mouth, she will find her spoon easier to use and will begin to enjoy feeding herself with it. Her attempts, however messy, should always be encouraged, but do not stop her from putting down the spoon and using her hands if she wants to. The most important lesson for her to learn is to enjoy her food.

You will of course want to be sure that your child is getting enough to eat, and it will sometimes seem that more food is sliding off the spoon than is completing the long journey to her mouth. Remember, though, that she will be just as anxious as you are that she gets enough to eat, and will certainly ask for more if she is still hungry when her bowl is empty. The answer may be simply to serve her with larger portions for a while to allow for wastage, or you can try making her blended meals with a bit less liquid so that the stiffer mix stays on the spoon more easily.

Always be ready to feed her yourself if she wants you to do so. Although she will enjoy feeding herself, the caring interaction of being spoon-fed by her parents is also important to her, just as the intimate contact of breast- or bottle-feeding was. In this as in other areas of child care, her parents' premature enforcement of her independence will be felt by the child as rejection, and will result in her prolonged need for reassurance. If you insist that she always feeds herself before she is ready to do so, you are much more likely to end up with a four-year-old clamouring to be fed than if you let *her* decide when she no longer needs your help.

The End of Weaning

Weaning is a process, not an event. But as your baby's appetite for solids increases, her enthusiasm and need for milk will slowly diminish, and eventually it will cease altogether. At some point in the second half of your baby's first year you may begin to offer a cup of milk after her midday meal, in place of her regular breast- or bottle-feed. If she accepts this, you and she are on your way to the completion of her weaning. If you have been breast-feeding, your breasts may be slightly sore for a couple of days, until your milk production drops to match the new, lower level of demand. Ending breast-feeding abruptly will be traumatic for your child and the pooling of unused milk is likely to cause you extreme discomfort. But a gradual reduction of the number of feeds given each day, whether from breast or bottle, should make it easier for both of you to complete the weaning. Some children take to the cup early and with glee; others need the comfort of bottle or breast for longer. But there is no 'right' time to complete weaning. It is a process which you and your child must negotiate between you.

At some point, though, you will probably be down to an early morning feed when your child wakes, and an evening feed just before she goes to bed. And the bedtime feed, because it calms and settles her for sleep, is likely to be the one she holds on to longest. There does come a moment when there is the last feed, the last bottle of milk, the point from which there is no return, whether it is you or your child who actually makes the decision. Inevitably this moment will evoke many painful and conflicting feelings in you both, as the completion of weaning marks the end of babyhood, and is a large step in the gradual separation between you and your child. Both of you may mourn the change, and she may be unsettled for a few days. But she will also enjoy her new-found independence, and you too will be able to celebrate as you watch her confidently making her way in the world.

Health Problems

Allergies   Specific foods can provoke an allergic reaction in some children, and those with a history of allergies in the family are especially likely to be susceptible. Cow's milk and cow's milk products (see page 73), the gluten contained in all wheat and wheat flour products and to a lesser extent in some other cereals (see page 41), and eggs, are among the most common food allergens. Allergies to soya milk, citrus fruits, tomatoes and fish are far from rare. A child's tolerance of these foods may grow as she gets older. There is some evidence that a lifelong allergy to certain foods can be triggered by their premature introduction to a child's diet. Certainly wheat and the other cereals containing gluten should be avoided until a child is six months old.

If a particular food causes an allergic reaction, withdraw it completely for a couple of months. Introducing new foods one at a time helps to identify possible problem foods. Allergic symptoms include streaming nose and eyes, wheezes, eczema, itchy rashes or weals, and frothy stools. In particular, a baby with a tendency to eczema may show a marked improvement if she (or, if she is breast-feeding, her mother) is taken off all cow's milk products.

If there is a history of allergies in the family, then leave not just wheat but cow's milk, eggs and citrus fruits too until the child is six months old, fish until she is nine months, poultry until she is a year. Give red meat with caution, if it is not excluded altogether. Take special care to avoid foods containing colourings, preservatives and flavourings.

Foods are by no means the only allergens, but a pure – and, as far as possible, an organic – diet should increase a child's tolerance to any specific allergen by reducing the background level of alien substances with which her body has to deal. Symptoms are more likely to appear, or will worsen, under stress, for instance during illness or when a child is otherwise disturbed or upset.

Constipation   Young children can become constipated, but this should *never* be treated by giving them additional high-fibre foods. Fresh fruit and vegetables, pulses and whole grain cereals are all rich in fibre, and a diet based on these foods should keep a child free from constipation. Wheat bran, rice bran or oat bran will fill a child up without feeding her, can damage her delicate stomach lining, and are likely to make her constipation worse rather than better as they absorb liquid from her gut. No laxatives of any kind should be given.

Diarrhoea and vomiting Neither diarrhoea nor vomiting *on their own* are causes for serious concern. Make sure the child has plenty to drink to replace the lost fluids, and keep a careful eye on her. If she has diarrhoea *and* vomits, however, or if she seems to be in pain or vomits repeatedly, call your doctor immediately.

Vitamins Vitamin supplements should not be necessary once the child's solid diet is fully established, provided that you are offering her a variety of fresh foods, and they should not be used unless specifically prescribed by a qualified practitioner. Imbalances of vitamins and minerals brought about by the excessive use of supplements can themselves lead to health problems.

Weight Children differ widely in body shape, and each child's weight may *appear* to fluctuate with the spurts and plateaux of her physical development. Trying to *reduce* a child's weight is very dangerous; in extreme cases a doctor may recommend a reduced intake of food for a while, in order to hold the weight steady until other aspects of growth have caught up. But it is worth remembering that there is no statistical association between above average body weight in under-fives and obesity in later life. A child's appetite can also fluctuate to a surprising degree, but as long as she is offered sufficient quantities of a variety of healthy and attractive foods no child will starve herself, so do not attempt to enforce a 'normal' daily intake. Showing respect for the feelings which determine how much your child wants to eat will enable her to grow up with her instinctive relationship with food intact – the surest way to avoid weight problems in later life.

When your child is ill, try to be as flexible as you can, both in the food and drink you offer her and in the way in which you allow her to take it. This applies to bouts of painful teething as much as to more serious conditions. When ill or in distress, a child is likely to revert in behaviour to an earlier stage of development. She will need extra emotional care and physical comfort, and should be allowed to eat very much what she wants, when she wants it. She may want you to feed her 'like a baby', on your lap. If this is the only way she will eat, do not discourage her; she needs the strength she will derive from the food and from your concern if she is to overcome this setback. Always make sure that she has as much as she wants to drink.

If a child has to spend time in hospital, find out from the nursing staff what kind of food she will be given and how it will be served. A sudden change in diet can in itself pose a major challenge to a child's health, and familiar foods will provide comfort and reassurance in a strange and frightening environment. Your child will appreciate special food treats in such circumstances, but she will probably enjoy even more some perfectly ordinary favourite food made by you and brought to her from home.

5 Eating with Everyone Else

Communal Meals

From the first hours of his life, your child will have learned to associate the satisfaction of his most pressing need, the need to appease his hunger, with physical, emotional and social contact. The bonding between mother and baby takes place initially through the interactions of feeding, and is recognized as an indispensable element in the early care of a newborn child. Even in cases of extremely premature delivery, where the baby must be fed through a tube passed directly into his stomach, doctors now acknowledge that he will benefit from physical contact, which reassures him that his hunger is being satisfied not just by a disembodied mechanical process but by someone who cares for him.

Breast milk is the best food for a newborn child, but even his own mother's breast milk, expressed and bottle-fed, cannot nourish him in the same way as the shared activity of breast-feeding. The full benefits of breast-feeding can only be gained when the physical and emotional intimacy between mother and baby is allowed to unfold in the repeated rituals of the feed, naturally and at the baby's own pace. But however a baby is fed, his ability to derive full satisfaction and psychological contentment from his food will depend on the quality of the emotional and social contact with which he is held, touched, talked to and smiled at as he feeds. This is no less true as a baby grows older. There is no point at which a child suddenly ceases to make the crucial association between the comfortable rhythm of hunger and satisfaction and the protection, care and love of his parents. Throughout life, 'breaking bread together' remains a significant occasion, in which the mutual love of families and of groups of friends is demonstrated and felt.

As soon as you can, begin to include your baby in family mealtimes. As we have made clear, the relaxed social enjoyment of food is an important factor in the happiness and well-being of adults as well as of children, and both parents are likely at times to resent the disruption of their meals by the demands of their young child. Be as flexible as you can, and try to learn how to relax and enjoy your meals in the changed circumstances brought about by the arrival of a new family member. To include him in the central family activity of mealtimes, you may need to adapt your own habits. Cut up your food before you pick up the baby, so that you can eat with one hand while you hold him. Learn to eat with your 'other' hand, and be prepared to be fed yourself by your partner. Partners can share the holding of their baby at mealtimes, so that each gets a chance to eat freely.

The disruption of your eating habits, and the chaos into which the kitchen will inevitably deteriorate from time to time as your child learns to feed himself, are a small price to pay for his early integration into the social life of the family, and for his easy adoption of a straightforward and healthy attitude to food. You may occasionally feel like banishing him from the family table 'until he has learned to behave properly', but he will have no lasting desire to disrupt family occasions into which he is welcomed, and will learn to respect and imitate your table-manners far more quickly if you respect and encourage his first faltering attempts to do so, however messy they are.

When he is very young indeed, before he needs or wants solid foods of any kind, a child who has been included from the first in his parents' mealtimes will begin to show his interest in what they eat and in sharing with them the food that they share together. His eyes will start to follow the passage of dishes from hand to hand, and of spoons from bowl to mouth, and before long he will be reaching for cutlery and food. As he becomes increasingly aware of his mother's importance as the source of his food, he may want to feed her. He is not only exploring the link between hand and mouth and the fascinating way that solid objects can disappear from one into the other; he is also beginning to recognize that his mother's need to eat corresponds in some way to his own need to suck, and seeks to satisfy her hunger as she does his. So the intimate interaction of breast-feeding begins to pass into the wider social interaction of the family meal.

There can be no definite rules about the timing of the various stages of the transition from breast- or bottle-feeding, through first solid foods and eventual weaning, to full participation in adult mealtimes and the ability to cope with unblended foods. Children do not all develop at a uniform rate, either in physical strength and stature or in the acquisition of skills.

Each child takes a slightly different path and proceeds at his own pace. And in illness, or when otherwise upset, a child who has been feeding himself with cut-up solid foods may want to return for a while to blended baby foods. The important thing for every parent to remember is that their child is not engaged in a race, in this area of his life any more than in any other. If you hurry your child, if you constantly force the pace in order to 'get through' each stage of his childhood, you will make him frustrated, neurotic and depressed. Try to let him learn at his own speed, always giving him the opportunity to sample new foods, or to feed himself with a spoon or drink from an adult mug, but *never* insisting that he do so.

Learning by Example

Your example will be the most significant factor in shaping your child's food choices and his attitudes to food. Remember that your child has sharp ears and eyes, and 'antennae' which are finely attuned to every nuance of his parents' behaviour. He will certainly learn from your example, but he is much more likely to pick up the 'bad' example set by your unconscious attitudes, or by ingrained habits which you have tried to conceal from him, than the 'good' one given by your ostensible precepts and commands. A child whose mother suffers from anxiety about obesity is likely to have feeding difficulties himself. She may do all she can to persuade him to eat good regular meals, but he will sense her anxiety (will perhaps see her alternately starving and bingeing, or notice the way she eats secretly), and will respond with anxieties of his own.

Once a child is enjoying blended solid foods in a settled way, it will not be long before he wants to sample the strange-looking foods he sees you eating. Naturally you expect that at some point in his childhood he will be eating pretty much what you eat; what is not clear is how fast he should reach that point. Your child's blended foods must be nutritious, and sufficiently pleasant and varied in flavour for him to enjoy eating them, and they must be offered in large enough quantities to satisfy his hunger. At the same time, if there are foods you do not want him to have, then you should not eat them in front of him. Provided these guidelines are followed there is no danger of his graduating to adult foods too early, and you can allow him to determine the pace at which he makes the transition.

There should always be at least one element of the family meal which he can have as much of as he wants. Steamed vegetables make ideal first finger foods, and he is certain to have his own favourite. Lightly cooked carrot pieces are usually popular, and will taste even sweeter to him if they come out of the same dish from which you serve yourself. Lightly salted bread and cheese can also be shared from an early stage (provided neither acts as an allergen). His meals will probably consist for many months of a varying mixture of blended foods and finger foods, and you should be able to eat your own meal in relative peace while he ruminates on a lump of solid food, breaking off every so often to give him a few spoonfuls of purée from his bowl.

If you follow the recommendations for cooking methods made later in this chapter (see page 125) and the recipes given in the section at the end of the book, his food and yours will not be so very different anyway, even when he first starts to take solids. You will wash, peel and chop the same vegetables for his dinner as for the family meal. To start with, you will cook them separately with certain different ingredients. But as he gets older you will more often be able to cook them together, perhaps taking out a portion to be blended for him before the addition to your main meal of certain ingredients, or perhaps only before adding spices and seasoning. This will not only save considerable time and effort; it will also make his transition to adult foods easier, for he will already be to a great extent sharing his meals with the rest of the family.

Your example will also be valuable to him in learning to

distinguish between what can and what cannot be eaten. At the stage when their child seems to want to put everything in his mouth (just at the time when he is learning to feed himself and exploring new foods at mealtimes, of course) every parent worries that he will pick up and eat glass, stones, mud, or worse. By encouraging him to share his food with you, you will have laid an excellent foundation for this lesson. It is far more effective to let him try to feed you with stones and to *show* him that you do not like them than it is to try to *explain* that these are not to be eaten.

Table-manners probably concern parents far less today than they did just one generation ago. Mealtime behaviour is nevertheless an important token and expression both of the mutual feelings of family or household members and of the value they place on the food they share and the work involved in preparing it. Your example is, again, crucial. It will be difficult to persuade a child that his food and his mealtimes are enjoyable enough to warrant his breaking off from his play if he only ever sees his parents eating on the run as they rush from one activity to another, or if one or other of them is consistently absent from the family meals. If family meals as such take place only rarely (at Sunday lunchtime, for example), and the usual pattern is for each member of the household to prepare their own individual meals and take them away to be eaten in bedroom, study, workshop or television room, a child will see no reason why he alone should accept what you provide, or why he should sit in his high-chair to eat it. His high-chair will at any rate be an unattractive proposition in these circumstances: instead of a comfortable observation-post at the centre of a lively and bustling kitchen, it becomes a lonely castle tower in which he is gloomily confined each mealtime.

As your child begins to extend the territory of his curiosity and the absorption of his play deepens, and as he learns first to crawl and then to walk, he will grow increasingly restless. Toddlers are notoriously reluctant to sit still. The happiest and most relaxed family mealtimes will be unlikely to compete with the exercise of his newly discovered talents, and he will often want to get down before you feel he has eaten what he should (and often before you have eaten anything at all!). A child who is compelled to sit still in a frenzy of impatience for permission to leave the table will probably come to hate everything to do with mealtimes.

What a child requires is freedom and flexibility within clear and consistently maintained boundaries. As far as the question of 'getting down before he's finished' is concerned, the only 'rule' which needs to be clearly understood is that your child cannot take his meal with him. If he prefers to crawl into another room to play, allow him to do so, without letting his departure disrupt the rest of the household's enjoyment of their meal. He should understand that the meal-table is the only place in the house where meals are eaten, and that his absence does not destroy the warm, relaxed atmosphere of the family's meals. You need not worry that he will starve himself: if he is hungry, he will come back, and should be welcomed as he rejoins the meal.

Family meals, in which all members of the household participate, should take place as regularly and as often as possible. They provide the whole family, and children in particular, with a fixed point of shared enjoyment from which to go out and explore the world as individuals. Eating is too important an element in all our lives to be treated as a necessary evil to be squeezed in between or alongside the 'real' activities of life. Healthy eating habits and a healthy attitude to food can only be fostered in circumstances that provide the space for concentration on communal eating as a worthwhile activity in itself. Your child's diet, and his digestive system, will benefit from regular family meals; he will more easily find his place within the family, and will develop social skills which will enable him more easily to take his place within the wider society when the time comes for him to leave home.

Quantities

Parents are often worried that their child may not be getting enough to eat. The unconstrained development of a child's natural appetite provides the best basis for a healthy lifelong attitude to food. It enables the child to avoid the feeding difficulties which pursue so many children from childhood into adolescence and even adulthood, and to establish a healthy diet as he gradually takes over the responsibility for making his own food choices. The over-anxious parent disrupts this process by introducing powerful emotional factors extraneous to the child's real bodily needs, which may nevertheless have a determining influence on his attitude to food for the rest of his life. Never force a child to eat more than he wants. His food must meet *his* needs, and *he* must be allowed to determine what these are.

Loss of appetite may be an indication of coming illness and a child who seems to eat much less than usual at successive meals should be carefully watched, but unless he is refusing food altogether it is unlikely that there is anything seriously wrong. It is worrying and frustrating when the food you have carefully prepared is rejected, but if you are patient with him his appetite will usually pick up again after a few days. Do not reduce the quantities offered at mealtimes. Sometimes an apparent loss of appetite can have a quite different cause. If the size of a child's meals has not kept pace with the growth of his appetite, he may have come to need mid-morning and mid-afternoon snacks which have reduced his need for his main meals. Or if he is particularly active, he may just prefer to eat snacks as he plays rather than meals for which he must sit still. Think carefully about how much he eats as snacks, and try to shift the balance of his eating back towards mealtimes (see page 124).

Except in extreme illness, a child will eat what he needs. Your job is to provide him with a plentiful and varied diet of nutritious foods. For the first two or three years his appetite will be growing fairly rapidly, and it is important to stay ahead of it in terms of the size of his meals. Do not worry about waste at this point; his appetite, though growing overall, will fluctuate, and you will find that he often does not finish his meals. But this is as it should be. If he regularly finishes every meal you provide, this should be taken as an indication that you need to increase the size of the meals you make for him.

A child will generally leave you in no doubt when he has had enough to eat, turning his head away from the spoon or simply spitting out what you have given him. Do not scold him for this (how would you show that you did not want any more if you were being spoon-fed and were unable to talk?), but be sure that he really has had enough to eat. It may be that he simply does not like that particular food, or more often that it is not what he wants at that particular time. Always try to have an alternative of some kind available: perhaps some suitable part of your own meal.

Never throw away his food after the first refusal: a child will often appear to lose interest in his food altogether for some minutes, but then continue to eat with gusto. The first few mouthfuls of a meal sometimes set off an involuntary peristalsis in the intestine, leading to a bowel movement which may occupy his full attention for some time! Be patient, and wait until he is ready to resume his meal. Occasionally, if he is upset anyway, or while teething, he may only eat when sitting on your lap rather than in his high-chair.

Choice

Choice is a key element in our enjoyment of food. As adults, we are often able to decide not only what we eat, but when and where we eat it. For a child, the exercise of choice in relation to food is limited to aspects of eating we tend to disregard because we take our absolute control of them for granted, but which are extremely important to him: the size of his mouthfuls, the speed at which his mouth is refilled, the means of lifting food from his plate, the arrangement of food on the plate, and the combination of different foods taken at a mouthful. Give your child as much control as possible over these aspects of his meals from his first taste of solid food onwards. Allow him to enjoy his food in his own way.

Do not assume that your child's food preferences will mirror your own. To an adult, the taste of food is its principal feature, but for a young child its temperature and texture are often more important. His delicate mouth and stomach need food which may seem monotonously smooth to us, and the blandest flavours will make him purse his lips in surprise when he first tastes them. It is always a good idea to taste his food yourself, not just to check the temperature, but also to attune yourself to his food preferences.

Introduce new foods carefully, one at a time (see page 100). Starting with a light, bland milled cereal such as whole-grain rice flour, the repertoire of ingredients can gradually be expanded through vegetables, fruits and pulses, eventually taking in wheat and, if desired, eggs, dairy products, fish and meat. The first time a new ingredient is introduced – the first time you blend a piece of pear or banana in with his rice porridge, for example – he is unlikely to show immediate enthusiasm, and may even appear to dislike the new flavour. Give him a few minutes to think about it, and show him that you like the food yourself. If he demonstrates a clear distaste for a particular food on several separate occasions, leave it out of his diet completely for a month or two before trying it again.

Rejection of a meal can be disheartening for the parent who has prepared it, and you may feel (and even say) that 'he doesn't like my cooking'. But you should not assume that your child dislikes a particular meal or a particular food because he refuses it at a single meal. He may simply not want to eat at all at that time. If you have used a new ingredient, it may be that he is not yet ready for it. On the other hand, if you have used only tried and tested ingredients, it may be that he is tired of the limited range of flavours available in the food you have been giving him, and would appreciate the introduction of something new.

A child's favourite foods are often the very foods that his parents do not want him to have. Never forbid your child to eat a particular food altogether: if you have chocolate biscuits in the house at all it is because you eat them yourself, and he will quite naturally refuse to accept that what is right for you is somehow wrong for him. But you must demonstrate the limits within which certain foods are eaten: that biscuits, for example, are only eaten at certain times (mid-morning or mid-afternoon, perhaps), and then only in certain quantities. You must, of course, observe these boundaries yourself, and must make it clear to your child that they are not negotiable. Never allow biscuits to become a substitute for any part of a main meal, and never engage in bargaining by giving biscuits as a reward or withholding them as a punishment (see page 21).

Timing

Timing can be a crucial factor in the establishment and main-
tenance of a child's eating patterns. In very early childhood, it
is the timing and duration of feeds which constitute the changing feeding pattern negotiated between baby and breast- or
bottle-feeding mother. We have warned against attempting to
impose on a baby a feeding routine for which he is not ready
(see page 78), but at some point every baby's feeding settles
down to a more or less fixed number of feeds, which take place
at more or less fixed times of day. By the time a child is eating
solids, this will probably have become established as three
main meals each day, with perhaps one or two liquid feeds,
and the regularity of these meals and feeds will have become
important to him. As adults, we can override our internal clocks
without too much discomfort, but a child is not able to do this,
and you should try to give his three solid meals as far as
possible at regular times each day.

Adults are also able to override the pinch of hunger in a
way which children cannot. We can forget to eat, just as we can
eat past the point of comfort. But the stomach of a child has a
far smaller capacity than an adult's, and empties and fills more
rapidly, sharply defining the passage from satisfaction to hunger
and from hunger to satisfaction. One moment your child will
be playing contentedly, and the next he will be crying with
hunger. He will voraciously devour every mouthful of food,
and just as suddenly announce that he has had enough.

The size of his main meals will of course increase as his
appetite grows, but if you are sure that you are serving him
large enough portions at mealtimes, and he is still finding it
difficult to 'last' from one meal to the next, it may be that he
just cannot comfortably eat at one sitting enough food to keep
him going until the next mealtime. You will find that there is a
constant pressure to produce meals earlier and earlier, or that
you are giving him snacks to keep him happy 'until it's ready',
with the result that his appetite for the meal itself is often
spoilt. There is no absolute reason why he should not have four
meals a day instead of three, but this is unlikely to fit easily
with family mealtmes. A better solution is to give him regular

small but wholesome snacks (see page 124), *not* when he starts to get hungry just before mealtimes, but midway between meals.

Although a child cannot be distracted from his hunger for anything like as long as an adult, it is also true that he will feel it earlier if he is bored than if he is busy. As your child's mealtime approaches, try to keep him amused for as long as possible. Do not begin the mealtime rituals of washing his hands, tying on his bib and sitting him in his high-chair until his meal really is ready, and do not show him his bowl until the food is cool enough for him to eat. To do either will be likely to increase his frustration, and if he gets angry enough he will be unable to enjoy his meal when it does come. An adult can understand that 'it's just coming, five minutes', but for a hungry child 'now' is often not soon enough.

Timing is also important in relation to spoon-feeding. Until he can feed himself, your child is dependent on your help. Try to feed at his pace, rather than forcing him to eat at yours. You can add greatly to his enjoyment of his meals by neither hurrying him nor making him wait for each mouthful.

Food Ideas

There is absolutely no need for healthy, home-made children's food, made from fresh whole ingredients, to involve any complicated cooking. Although the recipes given at the end of this book include accurate measurements and detailed cooking instructions, many of them can easily be adapted to vary the quantities, ingredients, and even cooking methods. Once you are confident with the range of ingredients and the basic methods of preparation you may prefer to use the recipe section of the book simply as a source of ideas rather than as a handbook, or you may find that your own imagination, and your pleasure in cooking good nutritious food which pleases and satisfies your child, leads you to create new dishes of your own.

We have included some more complicated 'special' recipes, but we know that many parents these days do not have very much time available for daily cooking, which is after all one of the main reasons for the growing popularity of so-called 'convenience' foods, both for babies and for adults. Very few of the blended meals require the use of more than one pot and a blender, and for those that are adaptations of a family meal you will need only the blender (in addition to whatever equipment you would be using anyway).

The saving of time and labour are not the only advantages of keeping children's food simple, however. Simple cooking allows you to manage more easily the combination and balance of different foods, and the careful introduction of new ones, so that you can ensure a proper supply of all the necessary nutrients in your child's diet, and identify and omit at an early stage any food to which he reacts adversely. The use of a fairly well-defined range of foodstuffs, both for your child's meals and for your own, will save money, reduce waste and ensure a rapid turnover of all stored ingredients, minimizing the deterioration of fresh fruits and vegetables, dried goods and refrigerated foods.

The remainder of this section looks at healthy food ideas for each of the three main meals of the day and for snacks, and in the following section we will consider the basic preparation and cooking methods which can be used to put these ideas into practice.

BREAKFAST

From some time usually between six and twelve months onwards (although it can be earlier than this, and may be later), when your baby no longer wakes for a night feed, there will be a gap of around twelve hours between his evening meal and breakfast, and he will probably wake up already hungry each morning. As long as you are still breast- or bottle-feeding you may give him an early morning feed, but if not, and certainly once he is fully weaned, the swift, smooth delivery of a filling and sustaining breakfast can make the difference between a ragged, stressful start to the family's day, and a pleasant and relaxed one.

The nutritional priority for a child at breakfast-time is to eat a good helping of some carbohydrate-rich food, filling his stomach, gently raising his blood-sugar level, and delivering the calories to sustain him through the morning. This is the *theory* of all breakfast cereals, for whole cereal grains provide an ideal package of unrefined complex carbohydrate (see page 43). Unfortunately, most of the branded breakfast 'cereals' are in reality very far from this ideal: they are made from refined cereal flour, are 'popped' and 'puffed' to give an illusion of greater bulk than they really possess, and deliver the majority of their calories in the form of the simple carbohydrates of added sugar.

Shredded Wheat is one genuinely unrefined and unsweetened manufactured breakfast cereal which can be used to provide a healthy basis for a child's breakfast, but oat flakes, whole grain ('brown') rice and rice flakes, millet and millet flakes, and wheat flakes themselves (either plain or malted), can also be used as the cereal base for a healthy breakfast. Oat flakes (or 'rolled oats') are readily available in supermarkets, but avoid 'instant' brands; these are pre-cooked, which impairs their nutritional value, and ordinary oat flakes cook rapidly anyway. All other flakes and grains are widely available in wholefood shops (and now in some supermarkets too). We would not recommend the use of oats or wheat (either manufactured cereals or ordinary flakes) before the age of about six months, and you should watch your child carefully when you first introduce them. Both oats and wheat contain gluten, which provokes an allergic reaction in some children (see page 100).

Shredded Wheat does not need to be cooked, but all the grains and flakes we have mentioned should be cooked for children up to the age of five or six, when a full set of teeth and fully developed intestinal flora enable the digestive system to handle raw muesli-style cereals. Whichever cereal is used, it is important that it is cooked with sufficient liquid to produce a loose (but not sloppy) consistency when served. Cereals absorb a surprising amount of liquid for their volume, and if they do not absorb it when they are being cooked they will absorb it from the child's stomach, leading to constipation and possible damage to the stomach lining. As a rough rule of thumb, most cereal grains and flakes require at least 2 volumes of liquid to 1 of cereal in order to finish cooking dry. For children, therefore, a ratio of *3 volumes liquid to 1 volume cereal* will serve as a basis, which may need to be adjusted for different cereals or to suit individual children.

It is quite unnecessary to sweeten any of these cereals with sugar, honey, or any other sweetener. However, the addition of fruit, either fresh or dried and rehydrated, does sweeten the food, as well as adding valuable vitamins and minerals and providing different flavours to vary the breakfast meal from day to day. Bananas and (peeled) pears are good fresh fruits to start with (before six months), and raisins and Hunza apricots (which must be pitted before blending) are good dried fruits. All dried fruits should be soaked for twenty-four hours, or overnight at least, to rehydrate before blending. Prunes and ordinary dried apricots (preferably unsulphured) can also be used and are effective if a child becomes constipated, but not more than one of either should be given in a single meal. After six months, nuts and seeds may also be added, and will improve the nutritional value of the meal. Almonds, cashew nuts, sesame and pumpkin seeds are all suitable, but it is important to make sure that no chunks are left whole on which a young child might choke; all nuts and seeds should be finely ground in the empty blender before other ingredients are added.

The liquid used may be milk (either cow's or goat's), soya milk, or formula milk, although it should not be necessary to use formula milk once a child is settled on three solid meals a day. If a manufactured whole-wheat cereal is being used, gently heat the liquid until it comes just to boiling point. Pour it over fresh or soaked dried fruit and any nuts and seeds (already ground) in the blender and blend until smooth, then pour the mixture over the crumbled cereal in the child's bowl and mix thoroughly with a spoon. If whole grain cereal flakes are to be used, add these to the cold liquid and slowly bring to the boil, stirring all the time. When boiling-point is reached, remove from the heat, cover with a close-fitting lid, and leave to stand in a warm place for five minutes before spooning into the blender with the fruit and blending as above, adding extra liquid if necessary.

As your child begins to enjoy finger foods and to share more of your food, you may find that he likes toast and perhaps eggs. A boiled egg can be given once or twice a week (but see page 38), and he can have as much wholemeal toast as he wants (although this should not be used as a vehicle for large quantities of sweet jam and marmalade). But continue giving him cereal porridge as his standard breakfast, varying the cereals and fruits used, for as long as he continues to enjoy it, as it provides the best possible food for the start of his day.

MIDDAY MEAL

There are advantages in making the midday meal the main meal of the day: a child is likely to be less tired, and will therefore be better able to concentrate on and enjoy his food in the middle of the day than in the evening. He may sleep better at nights if his heaviest (largest or richest) meal is not eaten late in the day. On the other hand, you may find that he is better able to sleep through the night if you *do* give him a large evening meal to sustain him through the long gap till breakfast. The shape of your day, and the timing of your normal family meals, will also influence the pattern you establish with your child.

There is no need to make your child's evening meal his main one simply because that is when you like (or are able) to cook, even if you normally eat only a very simple uncooked lunch yourself. If you follow our suggestion to freeze two or three meals for your child every time you cook for him, you can easily provide him with his main meal at midday by defrosting and heating a previously prepared meal from the freezer (or freezing cabinet of your refrigerator). You may find that your child shows no inclination to make either midday or evening meal his 'main' one, but that he simply eats as much as he feels like at each meal. You should certainly allow him this flexibility and it should present no problems to do so, provided you keep a stock of between two and six frozen meals – of two or three different kinds – ready at any time.

The midday meal will be based on a main dish, either frozen or freshly prepared, and we will discuss the preparation of these main dishes under 'Evening Meal', below. Try to avoid serving the same dish for both midday and evening meal: not only will your child appreciate the variety, but it is also difficult to incorporate the full range of nutrients in a single meal. Although a single dish can (and should) contain ingredients which either singly or in combination deliver some 'complete' protein (see page 42), vitamins and minerals will be derived from a range of vegetables, fruits and other foods, and the best way of ensuring the supply is to vary the ingredients used from meal to meal. Make the selection of dishes for midday and evening meals to suit your child: you may find, for instance, that a protein-rich meal containing meat or cheese is best served at midday rather than in the evening.

You will probably notice that your child's tolerance of (and need for) novelty of any kind tails off markedly as he gets tired towards evening. The later it gets, the more likely he is to seek the reassurance of familiar toys, games and rituals. This applies equally to food, and you will find that the midday meal is the best time to introduce new foods, extending the range of tastes and textures with which he is familiar. Remember that it is best to introduce new food ingredients one at a time, so that the cause of any adverse reaction can be more easily traced.

As he begins to experiment with finger foods, you may find that he likes to 'mix and match' for his midday meal, picking mouthfuls from an array of pieces of bread, cheese and fruit laid out on his tray. Always prepare and offer a hot main dish as the basis of his meal. Ideally, he will eat some or all of this before moving on to finger foods, but do not try to force him to eat it, or withhold healthy finger foods if that is what he wants.

Bread, rice crackers, cheese, soft raw salad vegetables (such as tomatoes and cucumber), *grated* cabbage and carrot, and peeled, pitted fruits (such as apples, pears, oranges and satsumas) all make ideal finger foods. Avoid salty cheeses, and try to vary the fruits and vegetables you give. Remember that until your child has most of his first set of teeth he will be unable to chew hard foods like nuts, some cheeses, and pieces of raw vegetables such as carrots, and there is a danger of his choking when he attempts to swallow such foods whole. Pears and oranges are usually safe enough, and he will manage most types of apple once his first molars are through.

There is certainly no need to provide a dessert at every mealtime. Your child will anyway not naturally distinguish between foods which you yourself would firmly associate with the different courses of a meal. He may, for instance, prefer to eat a bowl of puréed fruit *before* he starts on his main dish of rice and vegetables, or even to have the two mixed together! A simple, lightly sweetened dish such as blended cooked fruit or home-made custard (see the recipe section), although not necessary every day, varies the child's diet and can provide a useful source of vitamins, particularly for children who do not like raw fruit. Alternatively, half a banana or a peeled uncooked pear, mashed up with a couple of spoonfuls of cow's or sheep's yoghurt, makes a quick 'instant' dessert.

Stewed apples and pears make an ideal simple pudding, and if you have a freezer it is little extra trouble to make enough for many servings at one time. Choose eating apples, which will need little or no additional sweetening, rather than cooking varieties, which can be extremely tart if not sweetened with sugar or honey. Peel the fruit, or if it is organically grown or comes from your own garden, and you are going to use the skin of the fruit, wash it carefully. Core and roughly chop the fruit, and place in a pan with *very little* water. Lightly sweeten the fruit with honey or sugar if this is necessary; for pears, or even for a mixture of pears and apples, it will probably not be. Cover with a close-fitting lid, and simmer over a low heat just long enough to soften the fruit sufficiently to blend it to a smooth purée.

You can give your child as much as he wants to drink with his midday meal, either water or juice (see page 89). Cow's milk is a traditionally valuable source of protein, calcium and B vitamins for children, and can normally be introduced at around a year, or when the child has established a pattern of eating three full solid meals a day. Ordinary bottled milk should be used, and neither raw unpasteurized milk (which may contain bacteria with which a child is unable to cope) nor skimmed milk (from which the fat-soluble vitamins have largely been removed with the cream). However, cow's milk provokes an allergic reaction in some children, while others simply do not like it. In the case of an allergic reaction (see page 100), goat's milk can be tried as an alternative. Otherwise, you can either use a formula milk (if your child has already been drinking formula milk, continue with the same one), preferably given in a beaker and not in a bottle, or ordinary soya milk from a carton.

Both formula milk and ordinary soya milk must be used

with caution for the child who has just established his solid diet. Infant formula milk is designed as a sole food, and is richer in calories than a child who is eating three good meals each day really needs. Drinking a pint of formula milk every day on top of three solid meals may give your child more calories than he needs, and either make him fat or – more likely – impair his appetite for solid foods themselves. Look for a less rich 'follow-on' formula designed for the transition to solids.

Ordinary soya milk poses the opposite problem. It is useful as an ingredient in cooking for children who are not drinking cow's milk, but in itself when used as a drink provides much less nourishment than either formula milk or ordinary cow's milk: although its protein content is comparable with that of cow's milk, its content of vitamins and minerals (and of calories) is minimal. If neither cow's milk nor some kind of formula milk are being drunk, then once a child is weaned from the breast particular attention must be paid to providing sufficient calcium and sufficient vitamin B_{12} in the solid diet, whether soya milk is being used, or whether the child drinks only water and juices.

Many different brands and types of soya milk are available, and it is now widely sold in supermarkets as well as in specialist wholefood and health food shops. Several types contain added sugar (or malt) and salt, and there are also flavoured varieties. For regular use, choose from among the plain varieties, without salt or sweetening. You may prefer to use a brand made from organically grown soya beans, though this will cost a few pence more per carton.

EVENING MEAL

Detailed suggestions and recipes for main dishes are given in the recipe section, but we will try here to give an overview of the range of main dishes which are suitable for children from the time they have firmly established a pattern of eating three full solid meals each day, up to two and a half to three years old. Such dishes are equally suitable for either midday or evening meals, although as explained above a protein-rich meal which contains meat or cheese may be better given earlier in the day.

Until fairly recently, excessive consumption of carbo-hydrates was widely accepted as being the major dietary villain. This view is now largely discredited, and we know that in fact a diet based upon *complex carbohydrates* (see page 43) is likely to be much healthier than one in which carbohydrates are outweighed by protein. There is nothing wrong at all with thinking of your child's main meals in terms of 'carbohydrate plus other ingredients' so long as the carbohydrate element comes from an unrefined source, and one other than sugar. So, for example, you may choose one from a range of unrefined, mainly cereal, carbohydrate foods (which will probably include potatoes, brown rice, whole millet, wholemeal flour, wholemeal bread, and whole-wheat pasta) as the basis of each of your child's main dishes.

We will concentrate here on meals cooked on the stove top in a single pot. These have clear advantages from the point of view of convenience, and in fact there are very few meals which cannot be cooked in this way. The art of producing healthy, flavourful and varied meals using this cooking method lies in the timing of the addition to the pot of the different ingredients. Nothing is worse than the 'one-pot' stew into which everything has been bundled at the same time, so that one or two ingredi-ents will still not be properly cooked, when all the others have been reduced to a flavourless mush.

A further advantage of using a single pot relates to vitamin loss from cooked vegetables. All vegetables begin to lose their vitamins by exposure to air and light as soon as they are picked. Heat destroys an additional percentage of the vitamin content, but the traditional method of cooking vegetables by boiling drains most of the remaining vitamins into the cooking water, which is often tipped away. When cooking a meal in a single pot, all the liquid is used to achieve a smooth consistency when the food is blended after cooking, and the leached vitamins are therefore preserved. The vitamin content of the meal is maxi-mized if the vegetables are cooked only until just tender enough to be blended.

A typical meal might incorporate brown rice, lentils, pump-kin seeds, carrots, broccoli and tahini. Let us say that the meal is to be eaten at 6.00 in the evening. Brown rice takes between

40 and 45 minutes to cook. Normally, rice is cooked in just enough water (2 volumes to 1 of rice) so that it is all absorbed into the fully cooked grains. In this case, however, because we will be blending the meal for a child, we will need excess liquid at the end of cooking, and exact proportions of rice to liquid are not so important. So after rinsing it thoroughly in a sieve under the tap, at 5.00 we will add the rice, the carbohydrate basis of the meal, to about 3 times its own volume of water, in a covered pan over a high heat.

Green or brown lentils cook in 30 to 40 minutes. Red ones, which have been split, and have had the outer skin removed, cook much faster. In any case, we can add the lentils soon after the water has boiled, rinsing them first like the rice and, as for all pulses, sorting through them carefully to check that they are free of stones (see page 129). Once the water has returned to the boil we will turn down the heat to a gentle simmer, and will have more than enough time for the preparation of the vegetable ingredients.

All vegetables should be carefully washed in cold water, and carrots should be peeled if not organic or home-grown. Always buy 'dirty' carrots as opposed to washed ones. The bright orange carrots sold in supermarkets have been scrubbed, which increases the leaching of vitamins, and have been washed in powerful detergents which can leave an unpleasant soapy taste even after cooking. 'Dirty' carrots, whether organic or not, are always sweeter. Avoid chopping vegetables until just before they are to be added to a meal. Carrots take only 5 to 10 minutes to cook (depending on the size of the pieces) so we will not chop them until about 5.30 (which is also the time to add a small handful of iron-rich pumpkin seeds to the pan). At the same time we will chop the stalks of the broccoli, which we will add with the carrots at 5.35. The flowery heads of broccoli take no more than a few minutes to cook, and we will not add them until we are sure that all the other ingredients are cooked.

At about 5.45, all five ingredients should be ready; tender but firm and still full of flavour. Using a large mug or a ladle, we can now transfer the meal into the jug of the blender, filling it no more than three-quarters full. Be careful to distribute the cooking liquid evenly between the jugs of food if there is too much to blend at one time, if necessary adding further liquid (milk or soya milk) to each in order to achieve a smooth, loose consistency. Add a teaspoonful of tahini to each jugful. Using a spatula to guide it, pour whatever is not to be eaten straight away directly from the blender jug into clean, portion-sized freezer containers. Cover and seal the containers immediately, ready to go in the freezer (or freezing compartment) as soon as they have cooled. At 6.00, you should be ready to feed your child his meal.

This example is intended only to give an idea of the simple process of preparing not one but as many as *five* healthy main meals in a total work time of under one hour, and the ingredients have been chosen primarily for the sake of illustration. Further ideas are contained in the following section of this chapter, and in the recipe section at the end of the book.

Beware of giving your child too much to drink with his evening meal, as this can often cause disturbed nights when he wakes up wet. This is particularly the case if a bedtime drink is also given. Try offering a juicy fruit such as an orange, satsuma or tangerine as an alternative to an actual drink.

SNACKS
Snacks and snack foods often constitute one of the most critical and contentious issues in the negotiation between child and parent of the child's eating patterns. At their best, they complement a child's diet with simple, uncooked foods of the same kind used in his main meals; at their worst, they displace those foods with exotic but nutritionally inferior food treats.

For adults, snacks serve either to fill a gap of hunger left by the main meals or to satisfy a need for psychological 'nurturing' – for the feeling that food is 'special' – which the main meals have failed to meet. The healthy answer is to improve the quality (and perhaps also the quantity) of the food eaten at mealtimes, and to make mealtimes themselves more enjoyable. A child's stomach capacity is more limited, and particularly during spurts of rapid growth it is often impossible for him to eat enough at one meal to sustain him until the next. In this context, small healthy snacks given regularly midway between main meals are a useful way of bridging the gap. But it is very important that they are not allowed to become a *substitute* for good, satisfying and enjoyable meals.

If your child seems to need large snacks between meals, try to work out what is going on. If he regularly finishes all the food you give him at mealtimes, then you are probably not giving him enough, and should increase the size of his servings. If, on the other hand, he hardly touches his main dishes, so that he eats almost as much in between-meal snacks as he does at mealtimes, then it may be that what you are giving him is not sufficiently interesting. Try introducing one or two new foods, or increasing the proportion and the range of finger foods offered. At certain stages, it is natural for children to want to eat 'on the hoof': they are just too busy to want to sit down for long at mealtimes. But if your child consistently prefers to eat on his own rather than at the family table, then you should consider carefully whether your family mealtimes provide him with an atmosphere in which he feels comfortable and in which he can really enjoy his food. Mealtimes should be enjoyable highlights of his day, social events at which he is not simply fed but feels himself cared for.

Snacks should be of the same kind of food used in the child's main meals. Plain wholemeal bread, rice crackers, oatcakes and other simple unrefined cereal products, fresh fruit, raw vegetables and cheese all make easy and healthy snacks. Bananas, satsumas and other 'self-wrapped' fruits make particularly good snacks for journeys, although if bananas are regularly used as a snack food, they should not be given as part of main meals as well.

Manufactured snack foods will tend to undermine the healthy eating patterns which you and your child have established, and we would strongly recommend avoiding them completely (and this includes the new wave of 'health' snacks) at least for the first three years. By the time a child starts school, peer-group pressure and the pressure of advertising will certainly lead him to experiment with manufactured snacks, and a continued prohibition is likely to do more harm than good by turning them into 'forbidden fruit'. But your example, and the patterns established in his early years, will equip him as well as possible to make his own healthy food choices.

Basic Cooking Methods

We described in the previous section of this chapter, under 'Evening Meal', a simple method of preparing food in a single covered pan over a low heat, in which control over the cooking process is achieved by the timing of the addition of successive ingredients to the pot. This method may be used for preparing all your child's main dishes, but as he gets older you can vary the single-pot soups and stews cooked and blended especially for him with the introduction of elements of, or modified versions of, meals suitable for the whole family. This section contains brief descriptions of basic cooking methods useful in the preparation of the fresh, whole foods recommended in this book. It is really intended for the complete beginner, for the mother and father with little or no experience of using fresh ingredients in their cooking, but who wish to begin to incorporate these into healthy family meals which they can share with their child.

Vegetables

Most vegetables should not be boiled, other than in a one-pot soup or stew which will retain the liquid in which they have been cooked. They keep better colour, flavour and nutritional value if they are either *steamed* or *sautéd* (stir-fried). Cheap stainless-steel vegetable steamers are widely available in kitchen supply shops, department stores and some wholefood shops. They consist of a central base which stands on legs about an inch long, and surrounding 'petals' which open out to fit a wide range of pan sizes, the whole being perforated to allow the free passage of steam. Stand the steamer in a pan of water so that the level of the water is below the base of the steamer, and fill it with the prepared pieces of vegetable. Cover the pan with a close-fitting lid, and boil vigorously until the vegetables are just tender. Carrots, courgettes, all kinds of cabbage, cauliflower, broccoli and fresh beans are cooked ideally in this way, and can either be added to other ingredients in the blender for a child's meal, or be given as finger foods when cool. Several different vegetables can of course be steamed together. An ordinary metal sieve which fits one of your pans and will take a lid to cover the vegetables can be used in place of a proper steamer.

To sauté is *not* the same as to fry. Only a little oil is used, and the idea is to cook the vegetables in their own juices. All the vegetables mentioned above as being suitable for steaming may also be sautéd, as may aubergines (egg-plants), capsicums (red and green peppers), and all kinds of pulse or cereal sprouts. A light oil with a high smoking-point, such as sesame oil, should be used, and you will need a wide frying-pan (or a wok) with a fairly close-fitting lid. Alternatively, you can use an ordinary stainless-steel saucepan, though you will not be able to cook so many vegetables at the same time in this. Chop the vegetables into even pieces. Set the pan on a high heat, with just enough oil to cover the bottom. When the oil is hot (but before it starts to smoke) add all the vegetable pieces, and turn vigorously in the oil with a spoon or spatula. Leave the heat on a high setting and put the lid on the pan, removing it only to turn the vegetables with the spoon every thirty seconds or so. The vegetables should be cooked only until they begin to soften, and ideally should be served immediately.

Root vegetables, such as parsnips and swedes, potatoes, carrots and celeriac, as well as pumpkin, marrows and other squashes, are all excellent foods for the young child, either singly or in combination. Most are not suitable to be steamed or sautéed, however. Potatoes, parsnips and the squashes can of course be baked, but for a child's meals they are best boiled. Whenever possible boil them as part of a one-pot soup or stew, so that all the nutrients which drain into the cooking water are retained.

Cereals

Cereal grains have a central place in a well-balanced diet. They come in a variety of forms: whole, as flakes, ground into flour, and processed into a wide range of products, from bread to pasta. Rice and millet are the cereals most useful as whole grains when meals are to be shared with or adapted for a child. Both are gluten-free and may be introduced soon after a baby starts taking solid foods. Rice may be cooked in a one-pot stew but can also be cooked on its own, to be served separately to the adults and added to other ingredients of a child's meal in the blender, and millet is best cooked in this way. Choose an unpolished brown rice for general use, and if you want a white rice for an occasional change make sure it is a good-quality basmati rice rather than a highly polished commercial brand. Avoid branded pre-cooked rice, which is likely to be lacking in flavour and nutritional value. Rice is actually very easy to cook, and if you are only familiar with pre-cooked brands you will be surprised by the delicious flavour of the real thing. Millet, which is less well known, is a light cereal with a delicate flavour, ideal for babies; for adults it makes a pleasant change from other cereals, particularly in the summer when it can also be used in salads once cool. The following cooking method is suitable for both rice and millet.

Using an ordinary mug or teacup, measure the dry grains into a sieve, rinse them carefully under cold water and allow to drain. Rice and millet both swell to about three times their original volume when cooked, so one ordinary mug gives enough for two hungry adults (use the same mug each time and you will soon know how many measures you need). The flavour of both rice and millet is improved if they are briefly fried before water is added, so heat a little oil or melt a little butter – just enough to wet the bottom of the pan – and turn the drained grains for a few minutes over a high heat. The millet should begin to 'crackle', and you will smell the rice beginning to cook. Remove from the heat. Meanwhile you should have boiled a kettle of water. Now pour exactly *2 measures of freshly boiled water to 1 measure of rice (either brown or white) or millet*, and carefully add to the pan (if you have fried the grains as suggested the first measure of water is likely to bubble up as it touches the hot pan). Cold water may be used, but using freshly boiled water saves a little time. As soon as the water returns to the boil, turn the heat right down to a *slow* simmer, and cover the pan with a close-fitting lid. Do not stir at any stage, as this tends to break up the grains into a sticky mess. After 45 minutes, brown rice should be cooked, and should have absorbed all the liquid (40 minutes for millet, and about 12 for white basmati rice). A few minutes before this, push a fork to the bottom of the pan, and taste a few of the grains. If the pan is dry and the grains not quite cooked, add a little freshly boiled water; or if the grains are cooked, simmer with the lid off for a few minutes to boil off any excess liquid. Once cooked, stand the covered pan in a warm place for 5 minutes before serving. It is always better to season food with salt *after* it is cooked, but if rice or millet are to be used in a child's meal, then salt should certainly not be added until after the child's portion has been removed. Cooked rice or millet can be added to other ingredients in the blender straight from the pan to make a child's main dish, adding enough further liquid to blend the whole to a smooth consistency.

Cereal flakes are simply crushed whole grains. They contain most of the goodness of the original grain but with a dramatically reduced cooking time, and cook to a porridge rather than as separate grains. Brown rice flakes and millet flakes (both gluten-free) can be used as soon as a child starts on solid foods; barley and oat flakes (porridge oats), which have a small gluten content, can be introduced after six months. There is no particular reason to use wheat flakes; a child will normally be eating wheat in many other forms, so that it makes sense to vary the diet by using one of the other cereals for porridge. However, if there is no allergy to wheat, then wheat flakes too may be used after about six months.

Add 3 volumes of cold liquid for each volume of flakes in a pan. Plain soya milk is the best liquid to use for babies up to six months, when cow's milk may begin to be used. Alternatively, water can be used, but will make a blander, thinner and less sustaining porridge. Bring the mixture *slowly* to the boil, stirring gently with a spoon from time to time. When the porridge boils, continue to stir for a minute over a low heat and then remove from the heat, cover with a close-fitting lid, and leave to stand in a warm place for 5 minutes before serving. The flakes will continue to cook during this time, and you will in this way avoid the problem of porridge stuck and burnt on the bottom of the pan. For very young children, the cooked porridge will still have to be blended to achieve the smooth consistency they need.

Of the huge variety of flours available, ground whole rice is useful in the first few months of solid foods since it produces a smooth porridge without blending, and the basic method of preparing this baby rice from unrefined rice flour is given in the previous chapter (see page 90). Ground whole maize (maize meal) is also useful as the basis of healthy home-made custards (see recipe section).

Pulses

All the dried beans, peas and lentils are highly nutritious foods, perfectly complementing cereals to form complete protein when eaten as part of the same meal (see page 42), and are valuable as a regular part of any child's diet, whether or not he is also eating dairy products, meat, or fish. They can be introduced at about six months. All dried pulses except those which have had their skins removed – red lentils, and green and yellow split peas – must be soaked before cooking. Cover the beans with 3–4 times their volume of water (they swell to about 4 times their dry volume when soaked and cooked). If boiling water is used the soaking time can be reduced greatly, and black-eye beans will need only 1 hour of soaking, other beans about 4 hours. After soaking, *drain and rinse* the beans, and carefully sort through to check that there are no stones or other foreign bodies present. Sorting machinery in the countries of origin often allow through stones of the same size and weight as the particular bean, and these are more easily spotted after soaking, when the beans will have swelled. Cover the drained, sorted beans with about 3 times their volume of fresh water, and bring to the boil. Cover the pan, and simmer till cooked, when the beans should be not just chewable but soft, and with a floury consistency. Cooking times vary greatly, from less than half an hour for red lentils, up to 2 to 2½ hours for some of the larger beans. Cooked beans can be blended with other ingredients (usually including a cereal) in a child's main meal, or (in small quantities) can be given whole as finger foods.

Meat and Fish

Some meat can be introduced from about twelve months, fish a little earlier. As we have seen (see page 36), neither meat nor fish is strictly necessary for a healthy diet, but if you do wish your child to eat these foods, you will get better value for money (as well as giving him food of higher nutritional value) if you use fresh fish or good lean cuts of meat for one or two meals each week than if you give him supposedly cheap and convenient meat or fish *products*, such as pies, sausages, burgers and fish fingers, once a day.

All meat and fish must be stored, handled and cooked with great care, particularly for children (see page 48). To cook cod or haddock fillet for addition to a child's meal, heat a little oil in a wide frying-pan and place the fish skin-side down. Cover the pan and cook over a low flame for about ten minutes, or until the translucent flesh of the fish has turned white right through. Carefully remove the fillet from the pan with a spatula, and turn it over on to a clean plate. Using a couple of forks, peel the skin off the meat and discard. Now gently break up the fillet into flakes, carefully removing *all* the bones. A small quantity of de-boned fish (not more than a dessertspoonful per serving to begin with) can be blended with other ingredients for a main dish.

In general, meat should be stewed (boiled), grilled or roasted rather than fried, for children of all ages. Chicken stock, freshly made from the carcass of a roast chicken, and added to a child's soup or stew, is the best way of introducing meat, and small quantities of roast chicken itself can also be added to meals if the stock has been well tolerated. Small quantities of lean minced lamb or beef may be used later.

Taking Part

Activities surrounding the provision of the family's food are rich with opportunities for learning of the broadest kind. Whether his parents shop once a fortnight and cook a meal at home only two or three times a week, or whether they grow their own fruit and vegetables, cook three times a day, and make jams and pickles as well, a child will benefit from a full involvement in their efforts. As soon as your child can sit, allow him to participate when you are working in the kitchen. You will have to make sure that he cannot hurt himself, of course, but he can be happily occupied for long stretches rattling wooden spoons in a jug or sorting oranges from one bowl to another. He will enjoy the feeling that he is sharing in your activity, and it is surprising how soon this 'helping' becomes really helpful. If he can amuse himself for half an hour pulling all your pans out of the cupboard, then it will be considerably easier to allow him to do so while you get on with the cooking, and to clear up afterwards, than to spend that half-hour trying to keep him happy while preventing him from making a mess *and* doing your cooking!

Stacking, balancing, pouring and a host of other basic handling skills can be learned just as well playing with cooking ingredients and kitchen utensils as with special toys. When he can stand securely, pull a chair up to the kitchen sink and allow your child to 'help' with the washing-up. When you take him shopping, involve him in the selection of the different foods you buy, and if you do grow your own vegetables or fruit, let him see and touch the growing plants. Before long he will be able to take part in the preparation of the foods that he has picked, whether from a supermarket shelf or from a bush or tree, and will begin to make the connections, and to ask the questions, which will bring his imagination alive to the processes of nature and of human endeavour.

Away from Home

The older a child gets, the more often will he have to (or have the opportunity to) eat away from home. On family expeditions, journeys and holidays, when you are with him, try to provide a *similar* range of foods to the one he is used to, replacing fruit by fruit, carbohydrate by carbohydrate, and so on. Increasingly, however, he will spend time in the care of friends, grandparents and childminders, who may have very different ideas about food and feeding from yours.

Let the child find his own way. Neither he nor the person looking after him is likely to appreciate long lists of his likes and dislikes ('He just won't eat cauliflower but he *loves* asparagus', or 'He doesn't eat sweets'). He may surprise both you and himself by discovering new foods when he is with others, and the occasional day away from you, being spoiled with crisps and Coca-cola, chips and chocolate, is unlikely to do any permanent damage either to his health or to his acceptance of the more wholesome foods he is given at home. It is from his parents that a child acquires his fundamental attitudes to food. Your responsiveness to his needs, and the care you take over his food and your own, will have taught him to hear and heed the voices of his own tastes and appetite. Now you must allow him to exercise the right to make his own food choices.

6 Safety in the Kitchen

The kitchen is almost certainly the single most hazardous place in the home for children, so it is well worth considering and as far as possible reducing the risks before a child is old enough to be exposed to them. What we give here is a simple checklist of the most common hazards, together with advice on how to reduce them. This is not the place to give medical advice, but parents should know what to do in case of burning or choking, for example, as correct and prompt action can be crucial. If your child does have an accident and you are unsure what to do or how serious it is, *call a doctor or a hospital immediately.*

Burns Children can be badly burned by spills which an adult would hardly notice. Spilled cups of tea and coffee are a common cause of serious burns among young babies.

Never have a hot drink while you are holding a young baby on your lap, and take care not to leave cups of tea or bowls of soup near the edge of a table where a child could pull them over on to herself. Check deliberately every time you have to carry a hot pan from stove to sink or from stove to table that you are not going to trip over your child or over something she has put on the floor.

A tangle of electric leads is hazardous in any circumstances. An electric kettle with a lead which loops down from a work surface is a particular danger to a child, who may pull the kettle down on to herself.

Sort out your electrical appliances. Unplug and stow away any that are not in daily use. Make sure that the lead of an electric kettle cannot dangle below the level of the surface it is on. If this is not possible, unplug the lead at both ends when the kettle is not actually being used. Get into the habit of turning off power at the socket after using any appliance.

As soon as she can stand – even before she can walk – your child will probably be able to reach the handles of pans on the stove.

Stove-guards, adjustable for a range of cookers, are easily fitted and fairly inexpensive, and create a protective rail around the stove top. Even with a guard fitted, turn the handles of pans away from the room, and use the rear rings whenever possible. Be sure a child is well out of the way before you take something out of the oven – both your hands are likely to be occupied.

She may also be able to turn on the stove, particularly dangerous if you cook on gas.

Some cookers have controls well out of reach of a child. If yours is not of this kind, you may want to remove the knobs when you are not using the cooker. This is normally quite easily done using a thin screwdriver to lever the knob off its post. If you do cook with gas, be sure that boxes of matches are not left by the stove. If necessary, buy one of the spark-generating kind of stove-lighters.

Poisons Many quite ordinary household cleaners, which in many homes are kept under the sink or elsewhere in the kitchen, are highly toxic. Tobacco (if swallowed) and alcohol are also dangerous for young children, as are all drugs, which may be left in the kitchen if someone in the household takes pills at mealtimes.

You should know exactly what dangerous substances you have and where they are. Dispose of any that you are not going to use, and put the rest together in one cupboard. If this is within reach of an agile toddler (and very few cupboards are not) then you may want to fit a child-proof catch or an actual lock. Keep tobacco and alcohol well away from your child, and never leave pills on a table or counter where she may be able to get them.

Choking Choking can certainly be dangerous, even for an adult, but the danger to children from small objects is often exaggerated. Perhaps the children most at risk are those who have never learned to chew up or spit out lumps of food, because they have been unreasonably 'protected' from the risk of choking.

Until a baby is four to five months old she should certainly be given only liquids, puréed solids, or soft fruits such as bananas or ripe pears, but around that time (long before she has her 'chewing' teeth) you can start to give her small pieces of harder foods such as apple or cheese, and a bit later, toast. 'Mumbling' these between her gums will feel good to her, and she will learn early how to chew and swallow, and how to spit out what tastes or feels unpleasant in her mouth – a useful skill to have before she gets to the stage of picking up stones and buttons. Never give a child whole nuts (like cashews or peanuts) until her full set of teeth has grown in.

Knives Forks are probably more dangerous than knives to a very young child, who will not have the strength to cut herself seriously, even with a sharp knife. But all sharp or pointed implements are potentially very dangerous indeed.

Sharpened kitchen knives should definitely be kept somewhere where your child cannot get at them and put away immediately after use (bread-knives in particular are often left lying around where a child could reach them). She may like to have a completely blunt knife of her own (the shinier the better) so that she can 'help' cutting up vegetables. Let her hold and manipulate forks and unsharpened knives at the table as soon as she reaches for them, but only when you are there to supervise.

Falls High-chairs and 'booster' seats are invaluable (see page 95), but using them means that your child has further to fall.

High-chairs should have a good wide base if they are going to be at all stable, and a restraining strap between the child's legs to prevent her from sliding out under the tray. If a high-chair comes in several sections, as many do, the screws or bolts that hold them together must be checked regularly. 'Booster' seats should be securely strapped to the chair they are to be used with. Never leave a child sitting unsupervised in either high-chair or 'booster' seat unless she is firmly strapped in.

Fridges Children have been known to shut themselves inside large fridges and upright freezers.

If you have a fridge or freezer at floor level that is large enough for a child to get inside, fit a child-proof catch to the door. Chest freezers should be kept locked.

Recipes

Introduction

We have divided the recipes that follow into just two groups – recipes for special baby foods, and recipes for dishes which can be enjoyed by adults and children alike. The first includes meals suitable for babies from the time they start solids right through to two years old or beyond. The recipes in the second group have been designed to provide family meals, and the dishes can be given (with minor modifications in some cases) to babies and young children as well as to older children and adults. Where a recipe is not recommended for children below a certain age, we have made this clear.

The family recipes are scaled to provide two adult servings and one or more child's portions. Most of the baby recipes will yield two to four servings for a hungry toddler, and may therefore need to be scaled down during the first month or two of solid feeding.

Freezing   All recipes are suitable for freezing.

Fresh herbs   Many of the recipes call for fresh herbs. Dried herbs may of course be substituted where they are added during cooking (use a quarter to half the amount), but *not* where they are used as a garnish!

Salt   Very few of the recipes include salt in any form. Family meals can be seasoned after the child's portion has been served, or adults can add seasoning on the plate.

Shoyu   Shoyu and tamari are naturally fermented soya sauces, and contain valuable minerals. They also contain salt, and should be used with caution. A few of the recipes call for small quantities of shoyu. Avoid brands of soya sauce containing artificial flavourings and colourings.

Soya milk   Soya milk is used in many of the recipes. We mean unsweetened, unsalted and unflavoured soya milk.

Yoghurt   Similarly, we mean plain yoghurt. If possible, buy live yoghurt.

Baby Foods

APRICOT PUDDING
A sweet, textured baby dessert.

3 fresh apricots
1 dessertspoon pear juice concentrate
½ oz (15g) unsalted cashew pieces
½ oz (15g) sunflower seeds

Wash the apricots, remove the stones, and cut into small pieces.
Place the fruit in a pan with the pear juice concentrate and
gently simmer (covered) for 5 minutes or until the fruit softens.

Pulverize the cashew nuts and the seeds in a dry blender,
making sure no large pieces remain.

Add the softened fruit and all the liquid from the pan and
blend to a creamy consistency.

As an alternative to fresh apricots, 5–6 dried Hunza apricots can be used. Wash the fruit, cover it with water in a small
dish, and leave to soak overnight. The fruit should be soft
enough to use without cooking. Just remove the stones, and use
the water in which the apricots have been soaked instead of the
pear juice concentrate.

ASPARAGUS AND MILLET PURÉE
*If you are cooking asparagus anyway, why not allow your baby to share
in one of the most delicious treats of the year?*

1 level dessertspoon whole millet
5 dessertspoons water
1 spear of tender cooked asparagus

Wash the millet, then simmer (covered) with the water for
40–45 minutes over a low heat, without stirring. Blend with
the asparagus.

AVOCADO AND YOGHURT from 6 months

¼ of a ripe avocado pear
1 dessertspoon plain yoghurt
a squeeze of lemon juice

Mash all the ingredients together, and serve at room temperature. On its own, a little mashed avocado makes a wonderfully convenient food for babies from when they first take solids.

AUBERGINE AND POTATOE PIE

2 small new potatoes
2 teaspoons olive oil
½ a small aubergine (egg plant)
2 teaspoons lemon juice
½ teaspoon tomato purée
2 dessertspoons water

Scrub and boil the potatoes for 12 minutes or until soft.

Meanwhile, wash, peel and dice the aubergine in ½-inch cubes.

Over a low heat, warm the oil and turn the pieces of aubergine till they begin to brown, then add the lemon juice, tomato purée and water, cover the pan, and simmer for 5 minutes.

Mash all ingredients together.

BABY BORSCH

2 oz (50g) fresh beetroot (1 medium-sized beetroot)
2 oz (50g) potato (1 small potato)
2 oz (50g) carrot (1 medium-sized carrot)
a little soya milk

Peel the beetroot and the potato, scrub the carrot, and dice all the vegetables into even ½-inch pieces.

Place the vegetables in a small pan and just cover with

water. Bring to the boil and simmer (covered) for 15 minutes or until all are soft enough to cut through with a table knife.

Blend, adding enough soya milk to achieve a smooth consistency.

From 6 months, the soup can be served with a spoonful of yoghurt stirred into it.

BABY FISH DISH from 8 months

---

2 oz (50g) swede
2 oz (50g) potato
2 oz (50g) broccoli
2 oz (50g) fish (avoid oily fish such as mackerel)
1 teaspoon tahini
½ teaspoon lemon juice

Peel the potato and the swede, and wash the broccoli. Cut up all the vegetables into small pieces and steam for 10 minutes or until tender.

In a separate pan, steam the fish (or braise it in a little soya milk) until the flesh is white and flaky – about 5 minutes. On a plate, peel off any skin and carefully break up the flesh with a fork, making sure that you remove all bones.

Blend the fish with the vegetables, tahini and lemon juice, adding a little soya milk if necessary to give a smooth consistency.

BABY RICE

The best first cereal, made either from whole brown rice, rice flakes, or rice flour. The methods of preparation using whole grains and flakes are fully described in the text (see page 90).

Use a spoon – a teaspoon for a baby just starting on solids, a dessertspoon as appetite increases, to measure:

---

1 spoonful brown rice flour (ground rice)
6 spoonfuls plain, unsweetened soya milk

Whisk the flour and milk together in a pan. Bring slowly to the boil, stirring all the time. Remove the pan from the heat, cover it, and leave to stand for 5 minutes before serving.

BANANA AND PEAR
Smooth, sweet fruit, filling and tasty.

½ a banana
½ a ripe pear (peeled and cored)
¼ teaspoon lemon juice

Mash or purée the fruit together. Add the lemon juice to prevent discoloration if you plan to save some of the purée.

BROCCOLI AND SWEETCORN PURÉE
If you enjoy sweetcorn in season, this is a way of sharing it with a child too young to manage a whole cob.

---

a good-sized spear of broccoli
the corn of ½ a cob of sweetcorn

While the family's corn is bubbling in the pot, wash and chop the broccoli, including all but the toughest parts of the stalk, and place in a pan with 2 dessertspoons water and a squeeze of lemon juice. Cover with a tightly fitting lid and steam over a medium heat for 5 minutes.

When the corn is cooked, scrape the grains from half a cob on to a wooden board, using the back of a knife.

Liquidize the broccoli and the corn, adding enough soya milk to achieve a smooth, loose consistency.

CABBAGE AND SESAME SOUP

---

4 oz (100g) white or green cabbage
2 oz (50g) sesame seeds
a little soya milk

Wash and chop the cabbage, and place in a pan with 2 dessertspoons water. Cover with a tightly fitting lid and simmer over a medium heat for 5 minutes.

Meanwhile, grind the seeds in a dry blender.

Add the cabbage to the blender and liquidize, adding enough soya milk to achieve a smooth, pourable consistency.

CAMOMILE TEA

An excellent all-purpose drink from an early age, with a fresh, mild flavour. Don't sweeten it! Camomile is traditionally held to have soothing properties, and may help some children to cope with colic, teething, or other distress.

Herbal tea-bags are a bit more expensive but a lot more convenient than loose teas. Make up one tea-bag in a cup or pot, following the directions on the packet, and store in a sealed jar in the fridge. Dilute half and half with warm water in the bottle or cup when needed.

CARROT/BEETROOT JUICE

It is important that a child has plenty of drinks during the transition to solid foods. Freshly made vegetable juices are drink and food in one!

Wash, and if necessary peel, one or more fresh carrots or beetroot.

You may have a specially designed juice extractor, or a mixer with a juicing attachment. Alternatively, finely grate the vegetables on to a piece of muslin in a bowl, then gather up the cloth and squeeze out the juice.

Store the juice in a bottle or jar in the refrigerator, and serve diluted 1 part juice to 10 parts warm water to begin with, gradually increasing the strength to 1:5 by the age of 12 months.

Save the squeezed-out vegetable pulp to use in a soup.

CARROT AND PARSNIP SOUP
A sweet, thick, hearty winter soup.

---

4 oz (100g) carrots
4 oz (100g) parsnips
a little soya milk

Scrub or scrape the carrots. Scrub or peel the parsnips, quarter lengthwise, and cut out most of the woody (lighter coloured) centre. Chop carrots and parsnips into roughly equal 1-inch cubes, and place in a pan.

Just cover the vegetables with water, bring to the boil, and simmer (covered) until soft enough for a pointed knife to be poked into the pieces – 10 to 15 minutes.

Blend, using the cooking water and adding soya milk if necessary to achieve a thick but pourable consistency.

CARROT AND YELLOW SPLIT PEA SOUP from 7 months
A thick, rich soup.

---

2 oz (50g) yellow split peas
10 fl oz (275ml) water
8oz (225g) carrots
½ teaspoon brewer's yeast

Wash the peas and put with the water in a pan. Bring to the boil, then reduce the heat and simmer (covered) for 30 minutes.

Meanwhile, scrub or scrape the carrots, and cut into roughly equal 1-inch cubes.

When the peas are soft but still whole, add the carrot pieces and simmer (covered) for a further 10 to 15 minutes, until soft enough for a pointed knife to be poked into the pieces.

Blend, using the cooking water to achieve a thick but pourable consistency. Stir in the brewer's yeast before serving.

Cooking time can be reduced slightly if the peas have been soaked for a few hours beforehand – drain and cook in fresh water.

CAULIFLOWER AND MILLET SOUP
A lighter summer soup.

½ a medium-sized cauliflower
2 oz (50g) whole millet
8 fl oz (225ml) water
a little soya milk

Cover the millet with the water in a pan. Bring to the boil, and simmer (covered) for 30 minutes.

Meanwhile, strip any limp or discoloured leaves from the cauliflower and discard, together with the hard end of the stalk. Cut away the florets, and break into roughly equal pieces. Chop the remaining leaves and the soft core into slightly smaller pieces.

When the millet has been simmering for 30 minutes (it should be soft but still whole), add the cauliflower pieces and continue to simmer for a further 10 minutes.

Blend, adding soya milk if the cooking water is insufficient to achieve a loose, pourable consistency.

CELERIAC AND POTATO
This is a delicious variation on ordinary mashed potatoes, which you may find you like enough to cook it for the whole family!

2 small potatoes
4 oz celeriac
a little soya milk

Scrape or peel the potatoes, and peel the celeriac. Dice all into even ½-inch cubes. Barely cover with water, bring to the boil, and simmer (covered) for about 15 minutes or until tender.

Drain well, and mash with enough soya milk to make a creamy texture.

COURGETTE AND CASHEW PURÉE

2–3 small courgettes
1 heaped dessertspoon cashew pieces

The smaller the better! Courgettes more than about 3 inches long will have a tougher skin, and will need to be peeled.

Wash the courgettes carefully, trim the ends, and cut in half lengthwise. Place in a pan with 1 dessertspoon water. Cover with a tightly fitting lid and stew over a low to medium heat for 5 minutes.

Meanwhile, pulverize the cashews to a fine powder in a dry blender.

Add the courgettes with any cooking juices and liquidize.

CREAM OF WATERCRESS SOUP

A spicy new flavour to introduce after 6–8 weeks of solids.

1 small potato
1 small bunch of watercress
½ teaspoon lemon juice
a little soya milk

Peel and dice the potato and put in a small pan, barely covered with water. Simmer for 10 minutes or until it starts to soften.

Meanwhile, wash the watercress carefully, then chop, discarding the thicker stalks and any damaged leaves. Add the watercress to the pan with the potato and simmer (covered) for a further 5 minutes.

Add the lemon juice and blend with enough soya milk to achieve a creamy consistency.

FRESH FRUIT COMPÔTE

Fruit is a good source of vitamins and fibre, either on its own or mixed with a cereal such as baby rice. In the winter, when fresh fruit is scarce or expensive, use dried fruit (see Winter Fruit Compôte, below).

1 plum
1 satsuma
1 small or ½ large banana

Wash and stone the plum, and peel the satsuma and the banana. Blend all the fruit together.

WINTER FRUIT COMPÔTE

2 oz (50g) prunes
2 oz (50g) Hunza apricots
1 oz (25g) dried figs
1 oz (25g) raisins

Thoroughly wash all the fruit. Soak in a covered dish, well covered with cold water, for 24 hours. (Alternatively, use boiling water and soak overnight.) Remove stones from prunes and apricots, and any stalks from the figs. Blend with the water in which the fruit was soaked.

Give this dish to young children in small quantities, or mix it with plain baby rice to make a main meal. The concentrated fruit can cause an upset stomach if too much is eaten.

MELON AND CHERRY FRUIT SALAD

This is an excellent summer dish for a child just learning to eat finger foods. Roll up his sleeves and let him enjoy himself!

¼ of a ripe melon
2 oz ripe cherries

It is not always easy to pick a good melon. The end of the fruit should have the strong, sweet scent of the flesh. Ogen and Galia are good varieties.

Remove the seeds from the melon, slice the flesh from the skin and dice into bite-sized pieces. Wash the cherries, remove stalks and stones, and cut in half.

MILLET AND COURGETTE

A quick and easy main meal.

1 small (3–4-inch) courgette
¼ cup or 2 fl oz (50ml) millet flakes
1 cup or 8 fl oz (225ml) soya milk

Wash and trim the ends from the courgette. If the skin is not tender, peel it. Slice the courgette thinly and place in a pan with the flakes and the milk. Bring gradually to the boil, stirring all the time. Remove the pan from the heat, cover tightly and leave to stand for 5 minutes.

Mash or blend before serving.

MIXED VEGETABLE AND SEAWEED SOUP
Seaweeds are a rich source of vitamins, calcium and trace minerals, and are among the very few sources of vitamin B_{12}. Think of them as sea vegetables!

---

1 strip wakame seaweed
½ pt (275ml) freshly boiled water
1 medium-sized carrot
2 oz (50g) cabbage
2 oz (50g) frozen or shelled fresh peas

Put the wakame in a pan and pour over the freshly boiled water. Cover the pan and stand for 20 minutes.

Meanwhile, prepare the vegetables, slicing the carrot and the cabbage.

Add the vegetables to the pan with the wakame and bring gently back to the boil. Cover the pan, and simmer for 15 minutes. Liquidize.

NUT AND SEED MILK
A sweet, nutritious non-dairy milk drink. Not to be used as a substitute for breast or formula milk, but a good extra drink for the first months of mixed feeding.

---

1 oz (25g) cashew pieces
1 heaped dessertspoon sesame seeds
8 fl oz (225ml) water
1 teaspoon pear juice concentrate

Grind the nuts and seeds finely in a dry blender. Add the water and fruit juice concentrate, and liquidize.

PEA AND CAULIFLOWER PORRIDGE from 6 months

2 oz (50g) cauliflower florets
2 oz (50g) porridge oats
7 fl oz (200ml) soya milk
1 oz (25g) frozen or shelled fresh peas
2 dessertspoons peanut butter
½ teaspoon brewer's yeast

Cut or break the cauliflower florets into small pieces, and place with the oats in a pan. Pour over the soya milk, bring gently to the boil and simmer (covered) over a low heat for 7 minutes.

Add the peas and the peanut butter and simmer for a further 5 minutes.

Remove from the heat and blend to a smooth consistency, stirring in the brewer's yeast before serving.

PEA AND POTATO CREAM

1 medium-sized potato
2 oz (50g) frozen or shelled fresh peas
a little soya or cow's milk

Peel and roughly dice the potato. Half cover with water and bring to the boil in a covered pan. Turn down the heat and simmer for about 10 minutes, or until the potato begins to soften, then add the peas. Simmer for a further 3–5 minutes, then drain and mash or blend, adding soya milk or cow's milk to achieve a loose, smooth consistency.

PEACH MILLET COBBLER
An easy dessert or fruity breakfast dish.

1 ripe peach
¼ cup or 2 fl oz (50ml) millet flakes
1 cup or 8 fl oz (225ml) soya or cow's milk

Peel the peach, remove the stone, and cut into segments. Put the peach and the flakes in a pan with the milk. Bring gently to the boil, stirring all the time. Remove from the heat, cover tightly, and leave to stand for 5 minutes.

Mash or blend before serving.

PORRIDGE from 6 months

Traditional oat porridge makes the best cereal basis for breakfast from 6 months onwards. Before that, use Baby Rice (see page 90).

¼ cup or 2 fl oz (50ml) rolled oats (oat flakes)
¾ cup or 6 fl oz (175ml) soya or cow's milk

Mix the oats and the milk in a pan, and bring gradually to the boil, stirring. Turn off the heat, cover the pan, and leave to stand for 5 minutes.

Meanwhile, blend or mash a little fresh fruit.

Stir the fruit into the porridge, and serve warm.

POTATO WITH TAHINI

A filling savoury meal.

---

1 medium-sized potato
1 dessertspoon tahini (sesame paste)
a little soya or cow's milk

Peel and roughly dice the potato. Half cover with water and bring to the boil in a covered pan. Turn down the heat, and simmer for about 15 minutes, or until the potato is soft through.

Remove from the heat, drain and mash or blend with the tahini and enough soya or cow's milk to achieve a loose, smooth consistency.

PUMPKIN AND SUNFLOWER SPREAD

Cooked pumpkin is sweet and smooth, and an exciting bright orange colour!

About ½ lb (225g) pumpkin flesh
1 dessertspoon sunflower spread (or tahini)

Smaller varieties of pumpkin are sold whole, but the larger types are often sold by the slice. Whichever kind you buy, you will need a sharp knife to remove the tough outer skin. Scrape out the seeds, and if the pumpkin has been bought by the slice, cut away the outer layer of flesh which is likely to have dried out. Roughly dice the flesh, barely cover it with water and bring to the boil in a covered pan. Turn down the heat, and simmer for about 20 minutes, or until the pumpkin is soft through.

Remove from the heat, and mash or blend, adding the sunflower spread, and using enough of the cooking water to achieve a smooth, loose consistency.

QUICK RICE AND PEAS

1 dessertspoon brown rice flour (ground rice)
6 dessertspoons soya or cow's milk
1 oz (25g) frozen peas

Whisk the flour and milk together in a pan, and add the peas. Bring slowly to the boil, stirring all the time. Remove the pan from the heat, cover tightly, and leave to stand for 5 minutes.

Mash the peas into the rice before serving.

RICE, BROCCOLI AND ALMOND PURÉE

1 good-sized spear of broccoli
1 tablespoon brown rice flour (ground rice)
6 tablespoons soya milk
1 oz (25g) almonds

Wash the broccoli and chop it, including all but the toughest part of the stalk. Steam for 5–7 minutes, until the pieces of stalk are tender.

Meanwhile, whisk together the flour and milk in a pan. Bring gradually to the boil, stirring all the time, then remove the pan from the heat, cover tightly, and leave to stand for 5 minutes.

Pulverize the almonds in a dry blender. Add the broccoli and liquidize with just enough soya milk to enable thorough blending. Stir together with the rice.

RICE AND CHICKPEA SPROUTS

Beans, seeds and grains are easy to sprout at home. Eaten a few days after germination, sprouts are a valuable source of protein and vitamins, and are more easily digestible than before sprouting. Chickpea sprouts are especially sweet.

---

2 oz (50g) whole brown rice
10 fl oz (275ml) water
2 oz (50g) chickpea sprouts

Wash the rice, and cover with the water in a pan. (Using freshly boiled water from the kettle will save a little time.) Bring to the boil, then reduce the heat and simmer (covered) for 50 minutes.

Add the sprouts, and simmer for a further 10 minutes. Liquidize.

For a slightly older child, reduce the initial cooking time of the rice to 40 minutes, and roughly mash rather than blending.

RICE AND SPINACH WITH SESAME

One possible variation on the basic Baby Rice cereal (see page 142).

---

2 oz (50g) whole brown rice
10 fl oz (275ml) water
½ oz (15g) sesame seeds
2 oz (50g) fresh spinach
a squeeze of lemon

Wash the rice, and cover with the water in a pan. (Using freshly boiled water from the kettle will save a little time.) Bring to the boil, then reduce the heat and simmer (covered) for 55 minutes.

Meanwhile, toast the sesame seeds in a dry pan over a medium heat for 2–3 minutes, shaking the pan from time to time so that the seeds brown evenly.

When the rice is nearly cooked, wash and chop the spinach. Add the spinach, seeds and lemon juice to the rice, and simmer for a further 5 minutes.

Liquidize in the blender.

SWEET POTATO WITH MOLASSES AND TAHINI

1 medium-sized sweet potato
1 teaspoon molasses
1 teaspoon tahini

Bake the sweet potato in the oven as you would an ordinary potato, for about an hour at 375°F/190°C/Gas 5. (This dish is probably only worth preparing if you are using the oven anyway.)

When the potato is soft through, cut it open and scoop out the flesh. Mash together with the molasses and tahini, and serve warm.

Family Meals

APPLE AND BLACKCURRANT PIE from 7 months
A sweet fresh fruit pie with a savoury tang in the crust.

Make up a batch of pastry from the recipe on page 195, adding 2 oz (50g) grated cheddar cheese to the flour with the butter or margarine. Set aside in a cool place.

---

1 lb (450g) cooking apples (peeled, cored and sliced)
6 oz (175g) blackcurrants
2 dessertspoons honey
2 teaspoons apple juice concentrate

Mix all the ingredients together in a pan. Bring slowly to the boil over a low heat. Cover, and simmer for 3 minutes to soften the fruit.

Divide the pastry into 2 roughly equal portions and roll out into circular pieces, one slightly larger than the other. With the larger, line a greased 9-inch pie-dish, trimming around the edge of the dish.

Fill the dish with the fruit, and cover with the second piece of pastry, trimming and sealing around the edges, and making a couple of 1-inch cuts in the centre.

Bake the pie in the middle of an oven pre-heated to 400°F/ 200°C/Gas 6 for 35−40 minutes, till the crust is golden brown.

Any leftover pastry can be used to make Pastry Shapes (see page 195).

APPLE CUSTARD from 9 months – 6 months if the egg is omitted

a walnut-sized knob of margarine or butter
1 oz (25g) maize meal
10 fl oz (275ml) soya or cow's milk
1 egg (optional)
1 dessertspoon honey
1 eating apple

Melt the margarine or butter over a low heat, and stir in the maize meal thoroughly, using a wire whisk. Add the milk a little at a time, stirring constantly with the whisk, until a creamy consistency is reached.

Remove the pan from the heat, add the remainder of the milk, the honey and the egg, and blend together thoroughly with the whisk.

Peel and core the apple, grate it finely, and add it to the custard.

Return the pan to the heat and bring the custard slowly to the boil, stirring all the time. Simmer very gently for 5 minutes, stirring occasionally.

The custard can be served on its own or with other fresh or stewed fruit.

APPLE SAUCE

An easy and versatile dish: serve it hot or cold, with yoghurt and raisins, mixed into breakfast cereal, or as a side-dish with the Sunday roast! You may want to make it in larger quantities, to have a good supply available in freezer and fridge.

6 medium apples
a 1-inch piece of cinnamon bark or ½ teaspoon ground cinnamon
3 fl oz (75ml) water
2 dessertspoons apple juice concentrate

Any apples can be used, and if you have an apple tree in the garden this is an excellent way of using the windfalls. If you use eating apples, omit the apple juice concentrate.

Wash, peel and core the apples, and dice. Place in a pan with the cinnamon and the water, and the apple juice concentrate (if used). Cover tightly, and simmer over a low heat for 10–15 minutes, or until the apples soften.

Blend, using all the cooking water.

AUBERGINE SPREAD

An easy vegetable spread for a light lunchtime meal.

1 small aubergine (egg plant)
2 tomatoes
1 clove garlic (crushed)
1 dessertspoon lemon juice

Remove the crown of the aubergine. Grill whole for about 20 minutes, turning every 5 minutes, until it softens and collapses.

Meanwhile, dice the tomatoes into a bowl and add the garlic and the lemon juice.

Cut open the aubergine, scoop out the flesh and mash it together with the other ingredients.

Serve with warm wholemeal or granary bread, or with toast thinly spread with tahini.

BAKED APPLES

4 large Bramley cooking apples
2 oz (50g) raisins
4 good teaspoons honey
½ teaspoon ground cinnamon
4 dessertspoons water

Wash and core the apples, and score through the skin around their 'waists' with a sharp knife.

Place the apples in a baking-dish. Fill the holes in the apples with raisins, and spoon in honey until it overflows. Sprinkle cinnamon over the apples, and pour the water into the bottom of the dish.

Bake in a pre-heated oven at 375°F/190°C/Gas 5 for about 35 minutes, depending on the size of the apples. They will 'froth' when cooked, separating top and bottom skins.

BAKED BEANS from 7 months
These home-made beans are not just healthier, they're tastier than tinned ones too!

---

1 lb (450g) haricot beans
1 large onion
1 lb (450g) tomatoes
½ a red pepper
1 tablespoon olive oil
2 cloves garlic (crushed)
½ teaspoon chopped fresh thyme
1 teaspoon mustard
1 teaspoon sweet paprika
4 fl oz (100ml) water
2 dessertspoons honey

Soak the beans overnight.

Peel and finely chop the onion. Drain and rinse the beans, then put them in a pot with the onion and cover to twice their own depth with water. Bring to the boil and simmer (covered) over a medium heat for about 45 minutes, until just tender.

Meanwhile, wash and chop the tomatoes and the pepper.

Lightly sauté the garlic in the oil with the thyme, paprika and mustard for 2 minutes before adding the tomatoes, red pepper and water. Simmer for 5 minutes, then remove from the heat. Add the honey, and liquidize all in the blender.

Drain the beans, and mix them with the liquidized sauce in a casserole. Bake for 40 minutes in an oven pre-heated to 350°F/180°C/Gas 4.

Delicious served with Boston Brown Bread (see page 167) and perhaps a pork chop. Some children may prefer the beans mashed or even puréed.

BANANA FRITTERS from 9 months
Naturally sweet finger foods.

---

1 large or 2 small bananas
1 egg
2 oz (50g) plain wholemeal flour
1 teaspoon baking powder
3 fl oz (75ml) soya or cow's milk

Mash the banana, and beat in the egg with a fork. Mix the baking powder into the flour and combine with the banana and egg. Finally, add the milk and mix well.

Heat a skillet, griddle or frying-pan over a medium heat (and if necessary lightly coat the surface with margarine or butter). Use a dessertspoon to pour the batter on to the heated surface. Turn, to brown both sides.

Serve alone or with any fresh fruit, either hot from the pan or cold.

BANANA AND STRAWBERRY MILKSHAKE
A tasty and nutritious milkshake, without any added sugar!

---

1 dessertspoon sesame seeds
¼ of a ripe banana
2–3 strawberries
2 fl oz (50ml) soya or cow's milk

Grind the sesame seeds in the dry blender. Add the remaining ingredients and liquidize.

For variety, or when strawberries are not available, substitute half a peach or another soft fruit.

BASMATI RISOTTO

Unrefined brown rice is to be preferred to white rice for regular use. But the long-grained basmati has a specially delicious flavour and is much quicker to prepare than the brown, so use it for an occasional treat when pushed for time.

---

a good knob of butter or margarine
8 oz (225g) basmati rice – measured as 10 fl oz (275ml)
1 pt (575ml) water
1 dessertspoon olive oil
1 medium-sized onion
2 oz (50g) mushrooms
1 red pepper
2 tomatoes
3 oz (75g) frozen peas
a little freshly ground black pepper
1 dessertspoon shoyu

Melt the butter over a medium heat and pour in the rice. Stir for a few minutes till the scent of the rice starts to rise. Measure the water out of a freshly boiled kettle, and pour over the rice, taking care to avoid splashes as the water seethes. Turn the heat right down, cover the pan with a tightly fitting lid, and simmer very gently for 10–12 minutes, until all the liquid is absorbed. Do not stir the rice during cooking.

Meanwhile, peel and finely dice the onion, and wash and slice the mushrooms, red pepper and tomatoes.

Warm the oil over a medium heat, and gently fry the onion till it begins to soften. Tip in the prepared vegetables and the peas, and add the ground pepper and the shoyu. Cover the pan and stew for about 5 minutes, stirring occasionally.

Gently stir together the cooked rice and the vegetables in a casserole.

The risotto can be served immediately, but will be improved by baking (covered) in a pre-heated oven at 375°F/ 190°C/Gas 5 for 10 minutes.

Serve with a small knob of butter on each serving.

BEAN CHOWDER from 7 months

This is a lovely rich combination of fresh and dried beans, for serving with fresh bread and a green salad.

---

3 dessertspoons olive oil
2 medium-sized onions (diced)
¼ teaspoon cumin seed (ground)
1 teaspoon sweet paprika
3 teaspoons tomato purée
1 heaped dessertspoon tahini
10 fl oz (275ml) water
4 oz (100g) broad beans – from about 1½ lbs (700g) pods
4 oz (100g) previously cooked black-eye or pinto beans
2 heaped dessertspoons plain yoghurt

Warm the olive oil over a medium heat, and brown the onions with the cumin and paprika.

Stir in the tomato purée, tahini and water, then add the beans, cover the pan, and simmer for 5 minutes.

Stir in the yoghurt just before serving.

BEAN SALAD from 9 months

---

2 oz (50g) each cooked haricot and red kidney beans
1 Spanish onion (an ordinary onion will do)
2 tablespoons olive oil
1 tablespoon wine vinegar
1 teaspoon mild mustard (Dijon or similar)
1 teaspoon finely chopped fresh dill
1 fennel root
2 hard-boiled eggs

Dice the onion finely and add to the beans in a bowl. Mix together the oil, vinegar, mustard and dill, and pour over the onion and beans.

Stir together and put in the fridge to marinate for about 6 hours, turning every hour or so.

Before serving, add the chopped fennel and the sliced eggs.

BEEF RAGOUT from 1 year

This is a rich meat sauce for serving with potatoes, rice, wholemeal or ordinary pasta, or with 100% buckwheat noodles for a completely gluten-free meal.

---

2 medium-sized onions
8 oz (225g) rump steak
2 medium courgettes
4 oz (100g) French or runner beans
2 tablespoons olive oil
a little freshly ground black pepper
1 clove garlic (crushed)
1 teaspoon sweet paprika
1 dessertspoon tahini
1 dessertspoon tamari – similar to shoyu, but wheat-free
1 400g tin of plum tomatoes

Cut the onions in half lengthwise, peel them, and cut in slices widthways to form half-rings.

Remove fat and gristle from the beef, and dice into roughly ¼-inch pieces.

Wash the courgettes and the beans, top and tail, and slice or chop.

Warm the oil over a medium heat, and gently fry the onion till it begins to soften.

Throw in the beef, and add the ground pepper, garlic and paprika. Turn together until the onion browns. Stir in the tahini and the tamari, then add the tomatoes, courgettes and beans.

Bring to the boil, then reduce the heat slightly, cover the pan, and stew for 15 minutes.

BLACKCURRANT MUFFINS from 9 months

---

2 oz (50g) fresh blackcurrants
2 oz (50g) margarine or butter
4 oz (100g) or 3 fl oz (75ml) honey
1 egg
3 oz (75g) plain 81% or 85% ('brown') flour
1 level teaspoon baking powder

Allow the margarine or butter to soften.

Wash the currants and stew gently in a pan with 1 dessert-spoon water for just a few minutes until the fruit begins to break open. Set aside.

Turn on the oven to pre-heat to 350°F/180°C/Gas 4. Line a muffin-tin or tart tray with paper bun-cases. (This recipe yields 12 muffins.)

In a bowl, thoroughly stir together the honey and the margarine or butter, and then the egg.

Mix the baking powder into the flour, then add to the liquid mixture and stir for just long enough to reach a smooth consistency.

Spoon the mixture evenly into the cases – 1 good dessert-spoon each should work out about right.

Add about half a teaspoon of the fruit mixture to the top of each muffin, then place the tray near the top of the pre-heated oven and bake for 10–15 minutes. Test by pressing the top of the lightest muffin gently with your finger. If cooked, the muffin will spring back when the finger is removed.

Muffins can of course be made with a soft fruit mix made from any suitable fresh or dried fruit.

BLINIS from 7 months

Savoury buckwheat pancakes, entirely gluten-free. Traditionally served with caviar, you might prefer to try this recipe for a vegetarian alternative!

For the pancakes:
6 oz (175g) buckwheat flour
a little salt
2 eggs
12 fl oz (350ml) milk

For the filling:
2 oz (50g) carrots
6 oz (175g) spinach
6 oz (175g) mushrooms
a good knob of butter
½ a medium-sized onion (finely diced)
1 clove garlic (crushed)
1 dessertspoon tamari (similar to shoyu, but contains no wheat)
a little freshly ground black pepper
1 teaspoon lemon juice
4 oz (100g) cheddar cheese (grated)

It is best to make up the batter for the pancakes at least an hour in advance.

Put the flour and salt in a mixing-bowl. Make a well in the centre, and break the eggs into it. Using a whisk, gradually incorporate some of the flour into the eggs, then add the milk a little at a time, and carry on mixing until all the flour is worked into the batter. Cover the bowl and set aside in the fridge.

Wash and chop the carrots and the spinach, and steam them for 5 minutes.

Wash the mushrooms and slice them thinly.

Melt the butter over a medium heat, and gently fry the onion and garlic until the onion softens. Add the mushrooms, tamari, pepper and lemon juice. Stir together, cover, and stew for 7 minutes. Add the cooked carrots and spinach, and mash all together. Set aside.

Warm a wide skillet or frying-pan over a medium to high heat. When the pan is hot, melt a small knob of butter or margarine and coat the surface.

Use a very small cup to measure about 3 fl oz (75ml) of batter into the pan, and tip the pan to spread it to the edges. Turn with a spatula when the top surface dries out.

Take a good dessertspoon of the filling and lay it in a strip across the centre of the pancake in the pan, then roll the pancake around it. Remove the pancake from the pan and place it in a baking-dish. Repeat. (The recipe should yield 8 filled pancakes.)

When all the pancakes are cooked, sprinkle the grated cheese over them and place the dish under a hot grill until the cheese browns.

BOLOGNAISE SAUCE from 1 year

2 dessertspoons olive oil
1 large onion (diced)
1 teaspoon each finely chopped fresh oregano, thyme and rosemary
8 oz (225g) lean minced beef
4 oz (100g) mushrooms (sliced)
½ a green pepper (chopped)
4 tomatoes (chopped)
1 tin plum tomatoes
2 dessertspoons tomato purée
1 dessertspoon finely chopped fresh parsley
2 cloves garlic (crushed)

Warm the oil over a medium heat, and fry the onion with the herbs until it begins to soften. Add the minced beef and brown it with the onion. Add the mushrooms, pepper and fresh tomatoes. Drain the tinned tomatoes and add them, saving the juice. Add the tomato purée.

Stir all together and stew (covered) for 30 minutes. If the sauce seems too dry, add a little of the tomato juice at this stage. Stew for a further 30 minutes.

Add the parsley and the garlic, and cook for another 10 minutes.

BORSCH from 6 months – see also Baby Borsch (page 141).

---

8 oz (225g) beetroot
8 oz (225g) potatoes
8 oz (225g) carrots
4 oz (100g) cabbage
2 tablespoons olive oil
1 large or 2 small onions (diced)
½ teaspoon cumin seeds (ground)
1 teaspoon caraway seeds (ground)
1 clove garlic (crushed)
1 dessertspoon finely choped fresh chives

Peel the beetroot and the potatoes, and scrub or peel the carrots. Grate or finely chop all the root vegetables and the cabbage, and set aside.

Heat the olive oil in a large pan, and lightly sauté the onion and the seeds, adding the garlic.

Add all the other vegetables to the pan and pour over just enough water to cover them. Bring to the boil and simmer (covered) over a medium heat for 25 minutes.

Blend the whole mixture, or, if you prefer, leave about a quarter of the total unblended. Add the chives at the last minute.

Serve with a good spoonful of plain yoghurt in each bowl.

BOSTON BROWN BREAD from 7 months

A lovely sweet bread to serve with savoury dishes such as home-made Baked Beans (page 158). It has to steam for 3 hours, but it only takes 5 minutes to prepare!

---

6 oz (175g) wholemeal flour
6 oz (175g) 100% maize meal
1 teaspoon bicarbonate of soda
½ teaspoon salt
1 egg
4 fl oz (100ml) molasses
16 fl oz (450ml) soya or cow's milk
4 oz (100g) raisins

Sift the bicarbonate of soda into the flour and meal. Add the salt and stir together.

Beat the egg, add the molasses and the milk, and stir together.

Combine the dry and wet ingredients and mix thoroughly. The mixture should be sloppy.

Pour into 2 greased 2-pint pudding-basins (or equivalent). Divide the raisins, and sprinkle on each basin.

Cover the basins tightly with foil, and steam for 3 hours in 1 inch of water in covered pans, adding water as necessary to prevent them from boiling dry.

Run a knife around the bread and turn out on to a plate.

Serve warm with butter or margarine.

BUBBLE AND SQUEAK

More than just a good way of using up leftover potatoes, this is a delicious dish in its own right.

---

roughly equal quantities of cooked potatoes and cooked cabbage
a knob of butter or margarine
1 onion (diced)

Mash the potatoes, chop the cabbage, and mix thoroughly.

Melt the butter in a wide frying-pan, and lightly brown the onion. Tip in the cabbage and potato mixture, and press down into a flat layer.

Cook over a low to medium heat till a crispy brown crust forms on the bottom of the pan. Turn over and repeat 2 or 3 times.

BUCKWHEAT NOODLES AND FRIED VEGETABLES
Another simple gluten-free main meal.

---

an 8 oz (225g or 250g) pack of 100% buckwheat noodles
1 tablespoon olive oil
2 small onions (diced)
1 dessertspoon shoyu
a small piece of ginger root (grated)
2 oz (50g) mushrooms (sliced)
2 oz (50g) cabbage (chopped)
1 oz (25g) cashew pieces
2 cloves garlic (crushed)

Bring a nearly full pan of water to a rolling boil. Stir in the noodles and boil, stirring occasionally, for 7–8 minutes. Drain and rinse briefly under cold water. Keep warm.

Meanwhile, heat the oil and fry the onion for 2 minutes. Then add all the other ingredients and cook for a further 7–10 minutes.

Turn the vegetables with the noodles into a bowl and serve immediately.

CAROB BIRTHDAY CAKE from 9 months
Carob has the flavour of chocolate without the sugar and the caffeine, and is a good source of calcium.

---

2 oz (50g) raisins
½ a banana
6 oz (175g) margarine
12 oz (350g) or 8 fl oz (225ml) honey
3 eggs
8 oz (225g) wholemeal flour
3 heaped dessertspoons carob flour
1½ heaped teaspoons baking powder

Cover the raisins with hot water and leave to soak for 1 hour before baking.

In a large bowl, mash the banana, and mix thoroughly with the margarine and honey. Add the eggs and beat well.

Mix together the flour, carob and baking powder, and sieve into the bowl with the liquid ingredients. (Carob flour tends to go lumpy in storage.) Stir together for just long enough to achieve a smooth mix, then drain the raisins and fold them in.

Pour the mixture into two greased 8-inch sandwich tins, and smooth with a moistened spatula. Place in the middle of an oven pre-heated to 350°F/180°C/Gas 4 and bake for 25–30 minutes.

Test by pressing the centre of the cake gently with your finger. If cooked, the cake will spring back when the finger is removed.

Icing:

---

8 oz (225g) plain cream cheese
3 dessertspoons honey
1 dessertspoon sifted carob flour, *or* the grated peel of ½ an orange

---

Mix all together thoroughly. This will give just enough icing – either carob-flavoured, or with the contrasting colour and tang of orange – to fill and cover the cake. Happy Birthday!

CAULIFLOWER, MILLET AND FETA PIE from 6 months

2 oz (50g) whole millet
10 fl oz (275ml) water
½ oz (10g) sesame seeds
½ oz (10g) sunflower seeds
1 medium-sized cauliflower
2 dessertspoons olive oil
1 small onion (diced)
1 teaspoon ground coriander
2 teaspoons chopped fresh basil
6 medium-sized mushrooms (sliced)
1 dessertspoon shoyu or tamari
3 dessertspoons tahini
1 dessertspoon lemon juice
2 oz (50g) feta cheese

Place the millet in a pan with 8 fl oz (225ml) water. Bring to the boil and simmer (covered) over a low heat for 30 minutes.

Meanwhile, lightly toast the sesame and sunflower seeds in a dry pan over a medium heat.

Wash and divide the cauliflower into florets. Keep any undamaged leaves and the tender parts of the central stalk, and chop them into small pieces. Steam the florets and the chopped leaves and stalk for approximately 7 minutes, or until tender.

In a separate pan (you can use the one in which the seeds were toasted) heat the olive oil and add the onion, coriander and basil. Sauté over a medium heat till the onion starts to soften, then add the mushrooms and the shoyu or tamari, and cook together for 3–4 minutes.

In a bowl or a small jug, use a fork to stir together the tahini, lemon juice and 2 fl oz (50ml) water. Mix until it becomes smooth and creamy, then pour over the onion and mushroom mixture.

Add the onion and mushroom mixture, the cauliflower and the toasted seeds to the cooked millet and gently turn all these ingredients together before spooning into an ovenproof casserole.

Top the pie with crumbled or finely chopped pieces of feta

cheese, and bake (uncovered) in a pre-heated oven at 375°F/ 190°C/Gas 5 for 25 minutes.

CHEESY BROCCOLI from 7 months

---

16 oz (450g) broccoli spears
1½ oz (40g) butter
2 heaped dessertspoons wholemeal flour
10 fl oz (275ml) milk
4 oz (100g) stilton cheese (cheddar will do)
1 teaspoon sweet paprika
1 teaspoon mustard powder
1 dessertspoon chopped parsley

Wash and trim the broccoli, and steam for 10 minutes, until the stalks are just tender.

Meanwhile, melt the butter in a small pan, and thoroughly stir in the flour. Remove the pan from the heat and mix in a little milk at a time, using a whisk to disperse any lumps, until a smooth, creamy texture is reached. Mix in the rest of the milk and return the pan to the heat. Bring slowly to the boil, and simmer over a low heat for a minute.

Dice the cheese finely and add, with the spices and the parsley. Simmer the sauce for a further minute, until the cheese is melted.

Arrange the broccoli in a warmed serving-dish, and pour the sauce over it. Serve with boiled new potatoes.

CHICKEN PIE from 1 year

If you roast a chicken, don't just throw away the carcass. Any leftover meat can go into a chicken pie (which you may freeze for use later), and the carcass itself can be boiled with the bones to make chicken stock, which should be frozen immediately if it is not to be used straight away. Use the stock to enrich any soup or sauce.

Make up a batch of pastry from the recipe on page 195, adding a teaspoonful of crushed rosemary leaves to the flour. Set aside in a cool place.

---

3 dessertspoons olive oil
1 large onion (diced)
2 teaspoons finely chopped fresh tarragon
10 oz (275g) potatoes (diced)
10 oz (275g) carrots (diced)
15 fl oz (425ml) chicken stock
2 heaped dessertspoons wholemeal flour
8 oz (225g) frozen or shelled fresh peas
8 oz (225g) diced chicken
a little ground pepper
2 dessertspoons shoyu

Warm the oil over a medium heat and brown the onion with the tarragon. Add the diced potatoes and carrots, and turn with the onions for 2 minutes. Pour over the stock, bring to the boil, cover the pan, and simmer for 7 minutes.

Meanwhile, divide the pastry into two parts, one slightly larger than the other. Roll out the larger into a 12-inch circle, and use it to line a greased 9 by 1½ inch deep pie-dish (or similar). Prick the base well, and bake for 10 minutes in a pre-heated oven at 350°F/180°C/Gas 4.

Remove the pan from the heat, and stir in the flour. Add all the other ingredients, bring back to the boil, and simmer for a further 7 minutes.

Pour the filling into the pastry-lined pie-dish. Roll out the remaining pastry and cover the pie, trimming and pressing down carefully around the edges, and making two 1-inch cuts near the centre. Return to the oven for 35–40 minutes until golden brown.

CHICKEN SOUP from 9 months

---

2 medium-sized onions (diced)
4 oz (100g) cabbage
6oz (175g) potatoes
4 oz (100g) carrots
2 dessertspoons olive oil
1 teaspoon fresh tarragon (finely chopped)
1 teaspoon cumin seeds (ground)
4 oz (100g) lentils
30 fl oz (825ml) chicken stock
4 oz (100g) fresh or frozen peas

Peel and dice the onions, and clean and chop the cabbage, potatoes and carrots.

Brown the onions in the oil over a medium heat with the tarragon and cumin, then add the lentils and cook for a further minute. Add the prepared vegetables and pour over the stock. Bring slowly to the boil and simmer for 15 minutes. Add the peas and simmer for a further 5 minutes.

Blend half the soup and return to the pot before serving.

CHINESE STIR-FRIED VEGETABLES

If you run a busy restaurant in Beijing a wok is no doubt essential, but we find a good-sized stainless-steel saucepan a lot handier, and prefer our vegetables shaken, not stirred!

---

a small piece of fresh ginger root
4–6 spring onions
½ a red pepper
4 oz (100g) carrots
4 oz (100g) runner or French beans
4 oz (100g) baby maize
2 oz (50g) chickpea sprouts or mung bean sprouts
3 dessertspoons olive oil
2 dessertspoons shoyu

Peel the ginger root, ending up with a piece about the size of a chickpea. Slice thinly, then dice. Peel the onions and slice, including most of the green tops. Slice the pepper into thin strips. Clean the carrots and slice lengthwise into thin sticks. Top and tail the beans, making sure to remove any stringy edges from runners, then slice diagonally into thin strips.

Mix all the prepared vegetables with the ginger, the baby maize and the chickpea and bean sprouts in a bowl.

Over a high heat, bring the oil up to just below its smoking-point, then tip in all the vegetables and slam on the lid! With the heat up as high as it will go, fry the vegetables for 3–4 minutes (a little longer if the pan is really full), giving the covered pan a good shake every 30 seconds or so to turn the vegetables.

Pour the shoyu over the vegetables and serve with boiled rice.

COLESLAW

---

4 oz (100g) red cabbage (about ¼ of a cabbage)
4 oz (100g) white cabbage (about ¼ of a cabbage)
4 oz (100g) carrots
1 small onion (diced)
mayonnaise (see recipe on page 179)

Coarsely grate the cabbage and carrots into a mixing-bowl. Add the onion, and stir all together.

Make up the mayonnaise and stir into the mixture. Transfer to a clean serving-bowl.

COURGETTE PIE from 9 months

---

3 medium-sized courgettes
1 medium-sized onion
5 eggs
4 oz (100g) plain 81% or 85% ('brown') flour
1 teaspoon baking powder
2oz (50g) cheddar cheese (grated)
1 clove garlic (crushed)
2 teaspoons finely chopped fresh oregano
2 teaspoons finely choped parsley

Peel the onion and chop very finely. Wash and trim the courgettes and slice thinly.

Beat the eggs.

Combine the flour and the baking powder in a large bowl. Stir in the eggs, and then add all the other ingredients.

Pour the mixture into a 9-inch pie-dish and bake in an oven pre-heated to 350°F/180°C/Gas 4 for 45–60 minutes, until golden brown and firm in the centre.

Serve with boiled new potatoes.

COUS-COUS AND PINENUTS WITH SAUTÉD
VEGETABLES from 9 months

Cous-cous is a refined wheat product, but it is very quick to prepare and makes a good starch basis for a lighter summer meal.

---

2 courgettes
3–4 tomatoes
3 oz (75g) mushrooms
a knob of butter or margarine
6oz (175g) cous-cous   *a quick way of measuring is to use*
17 fl oz (475ml) water   *1 cup of cous-cous and 2 cups of water*
1 oz (25g) pinenuts
2 dessertspoons olive oil
1 clove garlic (crushed)
½ teaspoon sweet paprika
a sprig each of fresh basil and fresh parsley

Wash and prepare the vegetables, slicing them thinly.

Melt the butter or margarine over a medium heat and add the cous-cous and the pinenuts. Increase the heat slightly and turn the cous-cous for a couple of minutes.

Measure the water from a freshly boiled kettle, and pour over the cous-cous. Be careful, it may spit and bubble a bit!

Turn the heat right down, and stir the cous-cous until the bubbling has subsided and most of the liquid has been absorbed. Cover the pan, remove it from the heat, and stand it in a warm place. The cous-cous will be ready to serve in about 10 minutes.

Now heat the olive oil in a second pan, add the garlic and the paprika, and then the vegetables and the finely chopped sprig of basil. Cover the pan and increase to a medium heat, and sauté for 7–8 minutes, removing the lid to stir occasionally. If the vegetables appear to be drying out, reduce the heat.

Chop the sprig of parsley finely and add it to the vegetables for the final minute of cooking.

Fluff up the cous-cous with a fork before serving.

CRUDITÉS

This may sound fancy, but is really just a simple way of serving salad. Really fresh salad vegetables are often best enjoyed like this, and children will enjoy chewing on cool, firm and tasty pieces of vegetable.

Suitable vegetables to serve as crudités are carrots, celery, fennel, young courgettes, cucumbers, peppers (red, green or yellow), radishes and perhaps cherry tomatoes.

Choose young, tender vegetables, wash them well, and slice fairly thinly into pieces that will make a couple of mouthfuls. Prepare the vegetables as near as possible to the mealtime, and refrigerate until they are to be served.

Prepare little dishes of olive oil and/or mayonnaise (see recipe on page 179) in which to dip the crudités.

DHAL from 7 months

---

3 dessertspoons olive oil
¼ teaspoon each cumin, cardamom and mustard seeds (crushed or ground)
a small piece of ginger root (finely chopped)
1 clove garlic (crushed)
½ teaspoon sweet paprika
1 large onion (diced)
2 large carrots
4 oz (100g) cabbage
4 oz (100g) yellow split peas
30 fl oz (825ml) water
¼ of a red pepper
sprig of parsley

Warm the oil over a medium heat, and gently fry the seeds, the ginger, the garlic and the paprika for 1 minute, then add the onion. Cover the pan, reduce the heat, and cook for 5 minutes, stirring occasionally.

Meanwhile, scrub the carrots and dice small. Finely chop the cabbage. Wash the peas, drain and add to the pan with the onion and spices. Turn up the heat again and stir together. Add the carrots and the cabbage and fry for a further 2 minutes, stirring all the time.

Cover the contents of the pan with the water (freshly boiled from the kettle to save time) and bring back to the boil. Reduce the heat, cover the pan, and simmer for 35 minutes.

Finely chop the pepper and the parsley, add them to the pan, and simmer for a further 2–3 minutes. The peas should be starting to break up. Using a cup, transfer the contents of the pan to the blender jug and liquidize.

After a child's portion has been removed, the dhal can be further spiced with a little chilli powder or hot sauce. Serve the dhal with plain brown rice and a steamed green vegetable – spinach, runner beans, or okra – and perhaps with a side dish of yoghurt and grated cucumber (see recipe for Raitha, page 198).

EGG FRIED RICE from 9 months

Plain boiled rice left over from the previous day can be used in a number of ways – in salads, puréed with fruit to make a dessert, or fried up (with an egg if you like) for an easy hot lunchtime meal. See also Stuffed Cabbage Leaves (page 205).

---

1 oz (25g) sunflower seeds
1 oz (25g) sesame seeds
2 dessertspoons olive oil
1 medium onion
1 clove garlic (crushed)
2 cups cooked rice
1 egg

Peel and finely chop the onion.

Toast the seeds in a dry pan over a medium heat for 2–3 minutes, shaking the pan from time to time to make sure they brown evenly. Put on one side.

Over a medium heat, warm the oil and gently fry the onion till it begins to brown. Add the garlic and turn for a further minute.

Tip in the cooked rice, stir to break up the clumps, and mix well with the onion. When the rice is hot through, increase the heat and break the egg into the pan. Stir vigorously for 2–3 minutes.

Mix in the toasted seeds before serving.

EGG-LESS MAYONNAISE

Most mayonnaise, whether shop-bought or home-made, contains raw eggs, and should not be given to children. Here's a recipe that's completely egg-free.

---

2 fl oz (50ml) plain soya milk
½ teaspoon mild mustard
¼ teaspoon sweet paprika
¼ teaspoon salt
a little freshly ground black pepper
4 fl oz (100ml) olive oil
2 teaspoons lemon juice

Put the soya milk in the blender jug with the seasonings.

Now add the oil slowly while continuously beating the mayonnaise. If your blender has more than one speed, this should be easy. Run the blender on a slow speed, and very gradually pour the oil through the central hole in the lid. On single-speed blenders this can result in some messy splashes, so just add the oil a dessertspoonful at a time, blend thoroughly, stop the blender, add another spoonful of oil, and so on.

At this stage the mayonnaise should be creamy, but not thick. Add the lemon juice and run the blender for a moment at high speed, and miraculously the authentic mayonnaise consistency will appear!

Quite different flavours can be achieved by the addition of ¼ teaspoon curry powder, or of 1 dessertspoon very finely diced onion and 1 teaspoon tomato purée.

EGG SPREAD from 9 months

Boil the eggs at breakfast-time, and then this can be prepared in 5 minutes flat for lunch.

---

4 hard-boiled eggs
2 heaped dessertspoons mayonnaise (see recipe above)
½ a small onion (finely diced)
½ teaspoon mild mustard
a little freshly ground black pepper

Boil the eggs for 8–10 minutes, cool, and refrigerate if not to be used immediately.

Carefully peel the eggs, roughly chop them, and place in a bowl. Mash together with all the other ingredients.

FISHCAKES from 8 months

---

1 lb (450g) potatoes
1 lb (450g) white fish
1 oz (25g) butter or margarine
1 medium onion (finely diced)
sprig of parsley (finely chopped)
½ teaspoon sweet paprika
a little freshly ground black pepper
1 teaspoon mild mustard
1 oz (25g) wholemeal flour
1 oz (25g) sesame seeds

Scrub or peel the potatoes, and set to boil.

Meanwhile, warm a little oil in a frying-pan and gently fry the fish over a low heat for about 5 minutes, skin side down. Turn the fish on to a plate and remove the skin, then flake with a fork, taking care to remove all bones.

When the potatoes are cooked, mash them with the onion, parsley, paprika, pepper and mustard, then add the flaked fish and mash together well.

Mix the flour and seeds in a bowl. Form the potato mixture

into patties or fingers and roll them in the flour and seeds. Fry gently in a little oil until crisp and brown.

FISH PIE from 9 months

1¼ lb (550g) potatoes
1 lb (450g) fish – coley, haddock or trout
6 oz (175g) broad beans (from about 2 lb of pods) *or* 6 oz (175g) fresh or frozen peas
3 medium-sized carrots
½ a red pepper
2 dessertspoons olive oil
½ teaspoon coriander (ground)
knob of butter or margarine
1 heaped dessertspoon wholemeal flour
5 fl oz (150ml) milk
1 heaped dessertspoon grated parmesan cheese (cheddar will do)
8 oz (225g) shelled fresh or frozen prawns
2 hard-boiled eggs

Peel the potatoes (unless organic), and boil till soft enough to mash.

Meanwhile clean, wash and then dry the fish. Braise the fish for 5 minutes each side in hot oil in a wide, covered pan over a low to medium heat. Place the fish on a clean plate and break the flesh into pieces, carefully removing any skin and all the bones. Set aside.

Shell the beans or peas, and dice the carrots and the pepper.

Warm the olive oil over a high heat, and allow the coriander to sizzle for a minute before tipping in all the vegetables. Cover the pan, and sauté the vegetables for just 3 minutes, shaking the pan from time to time. Set aside with the fish.

Melt the butter or margarine in a small pan and thoroughly mix in the flour. Remove the pan from the heat and add the milk a little at a time, stirring with a whisk to disperse lumps, until a creamy texture is reached. Add the rest of the milk and the cheese, and return the pan to the heat. Bring gently to the boil, stirring continuously with the whisk, and simmer for 2 minutes.

Now put the fish, the vegetables and the prawns (which should be previously thawed if frozen) into a casserole. Peel the eggs, quarter them lengthwise, and then halve them across. Add the pieces to the casserole. Pour the cheese sauce over and gently mix.

Mash the potatoes, and spread evenly as a topping, smoothing down with the points of a fork.

Bake in a pre-heated oven at 350°F/180°C/Gas 4 for 1 hour.

FLAPJACK from 7 months

---

4 oz (100g) butter
4 fl oz (100ml) honey
2 tablespoons molasses
1 tablespoon malt extract
4 oz (100g) porridge oats (oat flakes)
3 oz (75g) wholemeal flour
2 oz (50g) raisins
1 oz (25g) dried apricots
1 oz (25g) currants

Melt the butter and mix with the honey, molasses and malt extract. Stir well.

Chop the apricots finely, then mix together with the oats, flour, raisins and currants.

Mix together the wet and dry ingredients and pour into a greased 1-inch deep baking-tin measuring approximately 7½ by 10 inches.

Bake in a pre-heated oven at 350°F/180°C/Gas 4 for 40 minutes, until firm to the touch.

GARLIC-ROAST PARSNIPS

This recipe has been known to convert confirmed parsnip-haters! It is good as an alternative to roast potatoes, or as a side-dish served with a thick winter vegetable stew. The pieces of parsnip come out crisp and chewy, and slightly sweet.

1½ lbs (675g) parsnips
about 2 dessertspoons soya oil
3–4 cloves of garlic, depending on size (crushed)
a little salt

This might seem like a huge quantity of parsnips, but there will be a certain amount of wastage and they do shrink during cooking.

Scrub the parsnips thoroughly. Cut away the tops, and any damaged parts. Quarter lengthwise, and cut into roughly even pieces about ½ inch square (cut the thinner pieces long and the fatter pieces short so that they cook evenly). Unless the parsnips are very old and tough, it is not necessary to remove the woody central parts.

Coat the bottom of a flat baking-dish with oil, and spread out the parsnip pieces. Add the garlic and sprinkle over a little salt.

Bake in a pre-heated oven at 375°F/190°C/Gas 5 for about 1 hour, turning the pieces of parsnip every 20 minutes to ensure that they cook evenly. They should be soft and just beginning to brown.

GOULASH from 1 year

1 lb (450g) potatoes
8 oz (225g) cabbage
3 large onions
6 rashers streaky bacon
2 dessertspoons olive oil
2 level teaspoons sweet paprika
½ teaspoon caraway seeds (ground)
2 teaspoons tomato purée
10 fl oz (275ml) water
1 dessertspoon tahini

Scrub or peel the potatoes, and dice into ½-inch cubes. Wash and chop the cabbage, and peel and dice the onions. Remove any rind from the bacon, and cut into 1-inch pieces.

Warm the oil over a medium heat, and fry the onion with the bacon, paprika and ground caraway till the onion begins to soften. Cover the pan and leave to stew for 5 minutes.

Add the potato, cabbage, tomato purée and water. Bring to the boil. Cover the pan again, turn down the heat, and simmer for 20–25 minutes. Lastly, stir in the tahini.

GREEK SALAD from 6 months

4 oz (100g) feta cheese, cut into ¼-inch cubes
12 black olives
2 spring onions (sliced)
4 large tomatoes (sliced)
4 oz (100g) cucumber (thinly sliced)
2 fl oz (50ml) olive oil
1 clove garlic (crushed)
½ teaspoon coriander seeds (ground)

Mix the garlic and the seeds into the oil and pour over all the other ingredients before serving.

Remove the stones from the olives in a child's portion.

GREEN SUMMER SALAD

6 leaves of lollo rosso (shredded)
1 ripe avocado pear (sliced)
1 large stick of celery (chopped)
1 bunch of watercress (chopped)
½ a green pepper (thinly sliced)
12 thin slices of cucumber
½ a punnet of mustard and cress
2 oz (50g) mung bean sprouts
1 oz (25g) alfalfa sprouts

Many children prefer salads which are undressed. For adults, this salad can be served with a dressing made by beating together the following ingredients:

3 dessertspoons olive oil
2 dessertspoons plain yoghurt
juice of ½ a lemon
1 dessertspoon finely chopped fresh chives

GUACAMOLE

Another simple vegetarian spread to serve with toast, with salads, or as a dip with Crudités (see recipe on page 177).

1 ripe avocado pear
1 small tomato
juice of ½ a lemon
½ teaspoon sweet paprika
1 small clove garlic (crushed)

Scoop the flesh from the avocado. Chop the tomato finely.

Mash all the ingredients together, and add a pinch of chilli after your child has been served.

HUMMUS from 7 months

An easy, protein-rich vegetarian spread from the Middle East. A tasty snack on wholemeal bread or toast, and a good accompaniment to salads in warm weather.

4 oz (100g) cooked chickpeas
3 dessertspoons olive oil
2 dessertspoons lemon juice
1 dessertspoon tahini
2 cloves garlic (crushed)
1 teaspoon sweet paprika

Liquidize all ingredients together in the blender. Garnish with sprigs of parsley to serve.

ICE LOLLIES I from 18 months

Save your children's teeth by making home-made ice lollies for the summer! The plastic lolly moulds (with reusable sticks) can be bought quite cheaply. Quantities in this and the following recipe exactly fill one type of mould, but check that yours have the same capacity and adjust the recipes if necessary.

2 good sprigs fresh mint
12 fl oz (325ml) water
2 dessertspoons pear juice concentrate

Allow the mint to steep in the water for 30 minutes. Remove the mint and mix in the concentrated juice.

Pour into the moulds, position the sticks, and place carefully in the freezer.

Substitute apple or blackcurrant concentrate for variety.

ICE LOLLIES II from 18 months

This one is more like ice cream on a stick!

6 fl oz (175ml) soft fruit
6 fl oz (175ml) plain yoghurt

Mash or purée the fruit (strawberries and bananas are easy and always popular) and mix with the yoghurt.

You can also use Apple Sauce for the fruit (see the recipe on page 156).

JERUSALEM ARTICHOKE SOUP

Another thick vegetable soup which can make an entire meal for a child.

---

8 oz (225g) Jerusalem artichokes
8 oz (225g) potatoes
2 medium-sized carrots
1 dessertspoon olive oil
1 large onion (diced)
2 cloves garlic (crushed)
1½ pts (825ml) water
sprig of fresh parsley (chopped)
½ teaspoon brewer's yeast

Scrub the artichokes and trim away any damaged parts. Boil them whole for 5 minutes, then drain and plunge them into a bowl of cold water. It should now be quite easy to peel them. Chop the peeled artichokes into ½-inch pieces.

Peel and dice the potatoes into ½-inch cubes. Scrub and chop the carrots into ½-inch pieces.

Warm the oil over a medium heat, and brown the onion with the garlic. Add the vegetables and stew (covered) for 2–3 minutes.

Pour on the water, bring to the boil and simmer (covered) for 20–25 minutes. Liquidize with the parsley.

Stir the brewer's yeast into the child's portion before serving.

KIDNEY BEAN MOUSSAKA from 9 months

There's no particular mystery or danger about red kidney beans, but like all the dried pulses they must be properly cooked.

---

3 oz (75g) red kidney beans
2 dessertspoons olive oil
1 medium-sized onion (diced)
1 teaspoon coriander seeds (ground or crushed)
1 teaspoon sweet paprika
1 small aubergine
2 oz (50g) mushrooms
2 tomatoes
2 oz (50g) French beans
2 cloves garlic (crushed)
2 fl oz (50ml) water
2 eggs
7 oz (200g) curd cheese

Soak the beans overnight, drain, and boil in fresh water for about 1 hour (depending on the size of the beans) until they are soft through. Drain.

Gently fry the onion and spices in the oil for a few minutes.

Wash and prepare the vegetables, roughly dicing the aubergine, mushrooms and tomatoes and chopping the beans into ½-inch lengths.

Add the garlic, aubergine, mushrooms and tomatoes to the onions, and stew (covered) for 15 minutes.

Add the French beans, the cooked kidney beans and the water, and cook for a further 10 minutes. Place in a casserole.

Beat together the eggs and the curd cheese, and spoon over the vegetable mixture as a topping.

Bake, uncovered, in a pre-heated oven at 350°F/180°C/Gas 4 for 30 minutes.

LAMB STEW from 1 year

1 large onion
2 teaspoons ground coriander seeds
2 cloves garlic (crushed)
2 dessertspoons olive oil
2 teaspoons fresh rosemary leaves (or 1 teaspoon dried)
3–5 lamb chops as required, depending on size
a little freshly ground pepper
1 dessertspoon finely chopped fresh parsley
6 tomatoes
8 fl oz (225ml) water
4 medium-sized carrots
1 large courgette

Dice the onion, grind the coriander and crush the garlic.

Heat the olive oil in a casserole, and sauté the onion, coriander, rosemary and garlic for 5 minutes over a medium heat. Put in the chops and brown on both sides, then add pepper, parsley, quartered tomatoes and water. Turn up the heat and bring to the boil.

Meanwhile, wash and chop the carrots and courgette. Add these when the pot comes to the boil, then cover and place in the middle of an oven pre-heated to 375°F/190°C/Gas 5 and cook for 45 minutes.

Serve with boiled new potatoes.

LEMON SOLE AND LEEKS from 8 months

1 lb (450g) leeks
6 pieces of lemon sole
½ pt (275ml) milk

Prepare the leeks carefully. Remove the root end and chop the white parts into ½-inch slices. Most of the green part of the leaves can be used unless the leeks are really old and stringy, but you will need to halve the green part lengthwise before slicing it, and then rinse it well to remove any grit between the layers.

Heat the milk to near boiling-point. Drain the leeks, then put them in a casserole. Lay the pieces of fish on the leeks, skin side up, and pour the milk over. Cover the casserole and bake in a pre-heated oven at 375°F/190°C/Gas 5 for 35 minutes.

Serve the fish carefully with a spatula, removing the skin and any bones from the child's portion.

LENTIL AND POTATO SOUP from 7 months

8 oz (225g) potatoes
2 oz (50g) cabbage
2 dessertspoons olive oil
2 small or 1 large onion (diced)
½ teaspoon coriander seeds (ground)
1 clove garlic (crushed)
4 oz (75g) red lentils
20 fl oz (575ml) water
2 heaped teaspoons tomato purée
2 teaspoons lemon juice
1 dessertspoon tahini
4–6 shoots of chives (finely chopped)
sprig of parsley (finely chopped)

Clean and dice the potatoes into ½-inch cubes, and wash and chop the cabbage.

Brown the onions in the oil with the coriander over a medium heat, until the onions begin to soften. Add the garlic and the lentils and stir for 1 minute.

Pour over the water, add the tomato purée and the lemon juice, and the prepared potato and cabbage. Bring to the boil, then reduce the heat, cover the pan, and simmer for 15 minutes. Liquidize.

Stir in the tahini and add the chopped herbs immediately before serving.

MEAT LOAF from 1 year

---

12 oz (350g) lean minced beef
1 medium onion
½ a green pepper
2 tomatoes
1 oz (25g) rolled oats
1 egg
½ teaspoon each finely chopped fresh chives, parsley and thyme
1 teaspoon mustard

Peel and dice the onion. Wash and finely chop the pepper and the tomatoes.

Using your hands, thoroughly combine all the ingredients in a bowl. Press the mixture into a greased bread-tin approximately 8½ by 4½ by 2½ inches. Bake in an oven pre-heated to 350°F/180°C/Gas 4 for 1¼ hours.

Serve with rice or potatoes.

MILLET PUDDING from 7 months

---

1 pt (575ml) milk
3 oz (75g) whole millet – measured as 4 fl oz (100ml)
1 tablespoon honey or maple syrup

Heat the milk to near boiling-point. Wash and drain the millet and put into a small ovenproof dish.

Stir the honey or maple syrup into the hot milk and pour over the millet.

Bake (uncovered) in the middle of a pre-heated oven at 350°F/180°C/Gas 4 for 45 minutes, stirring in the skin every 15 minutes or so. The pudding should be moist but not sloppy, and the grains of millet soft and fluffy.

MISO SOUP from 7 months

---

5 oz (150g) butter beans
4 oz (100g) carrots
6 oz (175g) cabbage
4 oz (100g) spring greens
2 dessertspoons olive oil
1 large onion (diced)
2 cloves garlic (crushed)
1 teaspoon each finely chopped fresh chives and thyme
2 dessertspoons miso

Soak the beans overnight. Drain, and boil (covered) in 2½ times their own depth of fresh water for 30 minutes.

Meanwhile, scrub and dice the carrots and wash and chop the cabbage and the greens.

Sauté the onion and garlic in the oil for 2–3 minutes. Add the beans and their cooking water, and the prepared vegetables and herbs. Simmer (covered) for 20 minutes, then remove from the heat.

Immediately before serving, take a cupful of liquid from the soup and stir the miso into it until thoroughly dissolved, then return it to the pot.

MIXED STEAMED VEGETABLES

Children enjoy eating steamed vegetables as finger foods, and this recipe gives a good mix of flavours to accompany fish or chicken. If you have only ever eaten onions fried or pickled, you are in for a pleasant surprise!

---

2 fennel roots
5 medium-sized onions
6 oz (175g) fresh young carrots

Trim the green stalks from the tops of the fennel, and remove any outer layers that are damaged or discoloured. Wash, then quarter lengthwise.

Cut the tops, but not the bottoms, from the onions, halve them lengthwise and peel.

Scrub the carrots and top and tail them. Halve lengthwise

any that are thicker than about ½ inch. Divide into 2-inch lengths.

Steam all the vegetables together for 12–15 minutes. They should be tender but firm.

MUSHROOM AND BUTTER BEAN PÂTÉ from 7 months

2 oz (50g) butter beans
2 oz (50g) mushrooms
1 dessertspoon olive oil
½ a small onion (diced)
½ teaspoon each finely chopped fresh basil and marjoram
1 clove garlic (crushed)
1 dessertspoon shoyu

Soak the beans overnight. Drain and boil for 1 hour in fresh water, until tender right through. Wash and slice the mushrooms.

Warm the oil over a medium heat, and fry the onion with the herbs until it softens. Add the mushrooms, garlic and shoyu and stew together until the mushrooms have cooked down.

Liquidize with the beans, using enough of the cooking water from the beans to achieve a smooth consistency.

MUSHROOM AND CELERIAC SOUP
Celeriac is a root vegetable with the delicate flavour of celery.

8 oz (225g) prepared celeriac root
4 oz (100g) mushrooms
1 large onion (finely diced)
a little freshly ground black pepper
1 teaspoon lemon juice
1½ pts (825ml) water

Because of its knobbly surface, there is quite a bit of waste when celeriac is peeled. Dice the peeled celeriac into ½-inch pieces. Wash and slice the mushrooms.

Warm a little oil over a medium heat, and lightly brown the onion. Add the mushroom slices and the pepper and turn till the mushrooms begin to soften. Add the lemon juice. Pour over the water and tip in the pieces of celeriac.

Bring to the boil and simmer (covered) over a medium heat for 35 minutes. Liquidize.

OATMEAL PANCAKES from 7 months

A fine alternative to the usual pancake batter, though cooked in the same way. These pancakes can be served warm, thinly spread with butter and honey, or used hot or cold as the basis of a variety of sweet or savoury dishes.

---

4 oz (100g) plain 81% or 85% ('brown') flour
4 oz (100g) fine oatmeal (oat flour)
½ teaspoon salt
10 fl oz (275ml) soya or cow's milk
5 fl oz (150ml) water
1 level teaspoon dried yeast
small knob of butter or margarine

Mix the flour, oatmeal and salt together in a bowl.

Warm the milk and water to blood temperature and stir in the yeast till fully dissolved. Pour the yeasted milk and water into a well in the flour and stir in with a whisk. Cover the bowl with a cloth and leave to stand for at least an hour.

Warm a wide skillet or frying-pan over a medium to high heat. When the pan is hot, melt a small knob of butter or margarine and coat the surface.

Using a very small cup, measure about 3 fl oz (75ml) of batter into the pan, and tip the pan to spread it to the edges. Turn with a spatula when the top surface dries out. Remove the pancake, re-butter the pan and repeat.

Serve straight from the pan or make a pile of the pancakes on a plate in a warm oven.

If you want to have pancakes for breakfast, you can make up the batter last thing the night before, using slightly less yeast.

PASTRY from 7 months

---

8 oz (225g) plain 81% or 85% ('brown') flour
½ teaspoon salt
4 oz (100g) butter or margarine
2–3 fl oz (50–75ml) water

In a large bowl, mix the salt into the flour. Using a couple of knives, cut in the butter or margarine until the mixture resembles breadcrumbs.

Add just enough water to combine all the flour into a dough that comes away from the sides of the bowl.

PASTRY SHAPES from 7 months
A simple and healthy savoury snack, ideal for parties.

Metal or plastic cutters can be bought quite cheaply in a variety of shapes: stars, trees, animals, and so on.

Make up a batch of pastry (see the recipe above), adding 2 oz (50g) grated cheddar cheese to the flour with the butter or margarine.

Roll out to about ⅛-inch thickness and cut out using shaped cutters.

Bake on greased baking sheets in an oven pre-heated to 400°F/200°C/Gas 6 for 7–10 minutes, until golden brown.

PEANUT BUTTER COOKIES from 9 months

---

1 egg
3 oz (75g) margarine
2 fl oz (50ml) honey
4 oz (100g) peanut butter
6 oz (175g) wholemeal flour
1 teaspoon baking powder

Beat the egg, and thoroughly mix with the margarine and honey. Add the peanut butter. Stir well. Sift together the flour and baking powder, and mix in.

Form into 1-inch balls and place with 2 inches between them on greased baking sheets. Flatten slightly with a fork to give a ridged finish. Bake in a pre-heated oven at 400°F/200°C/Gas 6 for 10–12 minutes.

These quantities give about 24 cookies.

PLAIN BOILED RICE

A nutritious and versatile staple.

Simmer 1 cup of brown rice in 2 cups of water in a covered pan for 40–45 minutes, until all the liquid has been absorbed. The method is described in greater detail in the text (see page 127).

PLUM SPONGE from 9 months

6 oz (175g) margarine or butter
6 ripe plums
12 oz (350g) or 8 fl oz (225ml) honey
3 eggs
9 oz (250g) plain 81% or 85% ('brown') flour
1½ heaped teaspoons baking powder

Allow the margarine or butter to soften. Wash the plums, remove stones and cut into quarters. Set aside.

Carefully grease a cake-tin, approximately 10 by 7½ inch rectangular or 10 inch diameter round, and at least an inch deep.

In a bowl, thoroughly stir together the margarine or butter and the honey, and then the eggs.

Mix the baking powder into the flour, then add to the liquid mixture and stir in for just long enough to reach a smooth consistency. Pour the mixture into the tray and spread to an even thickness with a moistened spatula.

Arrange the plum pieces evenly on top of the mixture, flesh side down. Place the tray in the middle of the oven pre-heated to 350°F/180°C/Gas 4 and bake for 25–30 minutes. Test by pressing the centre of the cake gently with your finger. If cooked, the cake will spring back when the finger is removed.

POPCORN

A healthy snack, always popular at children's parties. Plain, unprocessed popping corn can be found in most wholefood shops.

---

1 tablespoon oil
2 oz (50g) popping corn

Warm the oil over a medium heat. Tip in the corn, cover the pan, and turn up the heat. Holding the lid on tightly, shake the pan every few seconds until the corn stops popping.

Pour the popped corn into a bowl and sprinkle with a little melted butter or diluted shoyu.

POTATO PANCAKES from 9 months
Good finger foods, both freshly cooked and as a cold snack the next day.

12–14 oz (350–400g) potatoes (2 large or 6 small potatoes)
1 medium-sized onion
3 eggs
1 heaped dessertspoon plain flour
2 oz (50g) feta cheese

Peel the potatoes and the onion and grate them into a mixing-bowl. Add the remaining ingredients and mix well.

Remove enough for the child's portion before adding salt and pepper to taste.

Form into loose, circular patties between your hands and fry gently on both sides over a medium heat in a wide skillet or frying-pan, using just enough oil to coat the surface of the pan. Set on paper towels for a minute before serving to allow surplus oil to drain.

Serve with steamed green vegetables such as spinach, spring greens, or Savoy cabbage.

QUICK RICE PUDDING from 7 months
Here's a recipe for a simple pudding combining the virtues of whole grain rice and of speed – and it really is good, too! Wholefood shops stock the flakes, which are just crushed grains of whole brown rice.

---

1 pt (575ml) milk
3 oz (75g) rice flakes – measured as 6 fl oz (175ml)
2 dessertspoons honey

Set the milk to heat and stir in the flakes and the honey – use a small pot which can be put straight into the oven. (If you don't have a suitable pot, use a small pan and transfer the contents to an ovenproof dish at the next stage.) When the milk comes to the boil, place the pot in a pre-heated oven and bake (uncovered) at 350°F/180°C/Gas 4 for 20 minutes.

RAITHA
A cool, refreshing side-dish to serve in summer either with salads or with a curry or other spicy meal.

---

5 oz (150g) cucumber
4 oz (100g) plain yoghurt
2 leaves fresh mint (finely chopped)
1 dessertspoon lemon juice
a little freshly ground black pepper
½ a small clove of garlic (crushed very fine) – just a hint

Grate the cucumber and gently squeeze out the excess liquid with your hands. Place in a bowl and mix in the other ingredients.

Refrigerate until mealtime.

RASPBERRY FOOL from 7 months

---

12 oz (350g) raspberries
1 dessertspoon honey
5 fl oz (150ml) double cream

Wash the raspberries and mash them together with the honey. Beat the cream until stiff and fold the fruit into it.

Refrigerate until ready to serve.

RASPBERRY TOFU SLICE from 7 months
A sweet treat that is also a perfect protein combination!

For the base:
2 oz (50g) wholemeal flour
4 oz (100g) millet flakes
4 oz (100g) porridge oats (oat flakes)
8 oz (25g) or 5 fl oz (150ml) honey
4 oz (100g) margarine

For the topping:
8 oz (225g) raspberries
10 oz (275g) tofu
juice and grated rind of ½ a lemon
4 oz (100g) or 3 fl oz (75ml) honey

Mix together the flour and flakes in a bowl. Add the honey and margarine, and work together well. Spoon into a greased rectangular tray approximately 7½ by 10 inches and smooth with a moistened spatula. Bake in the middle of a pre-heated oven at 350°F/180°C/Gas 4 for 10 minutes.

Meanwhile, wash the raspberries and blend with the other ingredients of the topping to a smooth cream. Pour on to the pre-baked base, smooth to the edges and bake for a further 25 minutes. The topping should be set but soft.

Refrigerate any cake that is left over.

RATATOUILLE

1 large aubergine
2 large courgettes
4 tomatoes
3 dessertspoons olive oil
2 medium-sized onions (sliced)
1 dessertspoon finely chopped fresh chives
1 teaspoon each finely chopped fresh rosemary, marjoram and thyme
3 cloves garlic (crushed)
4 fl oz (100ml) water
juice of ½ a lemon

Wash and slice the aubergine, courgettes and tomatoes.

Sauté the onion and the herbs in the oil over a medium heat until the onion is tender. Add the slices of aubergine, courgette and tomato, and the garlic, and stir for 2–3 minutes.

Pour over the water, bring to the boil, and simmer (covered) over a low heat for 30 minutes. Add the lemon juice before serving.

RED CABBAGE AND APPLE

8 oz (225g) red cabbage, or ¼ of a cabbage
1 Cox's apple (or other eating variety)
1 oz (25g) raisins
1 dessertspoon red wine vinegar

Divide the cabbage into quarters, and remove the central stalk and any damaged or withered outer leaves. Slice thinly lengthwise. Peel and core the apple, and slice thinly. Wash the raisins.

Mix the cabbage with the apple and raisins in a steamer, sieve or colander, and steam (well covered) for 12 minutes or until the cabbage is tender. Pour the vinegar over and turn.

Serve with a knob of butter.

RED AND GREEN SPAGHETTI SAUCE

A quick and attractive vegetarian spaghetti sauce.

---

2 medium-sized onions
1 medium-sized carrot
½ a red pepper
2 tablespoons olive oil
2 cloves garlic (crushed)
½ teaspoon sweet paprika
1 14 oz (400g) tin of plum tomatoes
1 teaspoon tomato purée
4 oz (100g) spinach
a sprig each of thyme and parsley

Peel and finely chop the onions. Scrub and slice the carrot, and wash and slice the pepper.

Warm the oil over a medium heat, and gently sauté the onion with the garlic and the paprika for 3–4 minutes, until it begins to soften. Pour over the tomatoes and add the tomato purée. Turn up the heat and bring to the boil, stirring. Simmer vigorously, uncovered, over a medium heat for 10 minutes to reduce the liquid.

Meanwhile, wash and chop the spinach, and finely chop the thyme and parsley. Add the spinach and the herbs and simmer for a further 3–4 minutes before serving.

Serve with 200g of pasta for each adult and 50–75g for a child.

SAVOURY PUMPKIN PIE from 9 months

Make up a half-batch of pastry from the recipe on page 195

---

1 lb (450g) pumpkin
2 dessertspoons olive oil
1 large onion (diced)
½ a red pepper
½ a green pepper
a small piece of fresh ginger (grated)
½ teaspoon finely chopped fresh thyme
2 oz (50g) cheddar cheese (grated)
1 egg
1 tomato

Roll out the pastry into a circle and line a greased 9-inch pie-dish. Trim the edges, prick well with a fork, and bake in an oven pre-heated to 375°F/190°C/Gas 5 for 10 minutes.

Meanwhile, peel and cut the pumpkin into 1-inch cubes. Barely cover with water, bring to the boil and simmer for 10 minutes or until tender.

Wash and dice the pepper. Sauté the onion and the pepper in the oil over a medium heat with the ginger and thyme until the onion is tender.

Drain and mash the pumpkin. Stir in the sautéed vegetables and the cheese. Beat the egg and stir in thoroughly.

Pour the mixture into the pie case. Slice the tomato thinly and use the slices to decorate the pie. Bake at 375°F/190°C/Gas 5 for 25 minutes until golden brown.

Serve either hot or cold.

SCALLOPED POTATOES from 7 months

---

1 lb (450g) potatoes
2 dessertspoons wholemeal flour
3 dessertspoons grated parmesan cheese
1 heaped teaspoon sweet paprika
½ teaspoon ground pepper
½ a green pepper
1 oz (25g) butter or margarine
15 fl oz (425ml) milk

Peel the potatoes and slice thinly. Set aside.

In a small bowl, combine the flour, cheese and spices. Wash the pepper and cut into very fine slices.

Grease a casserole and make 4 layers of potato slices, scattering some of the flour mixture and some slices of pepper between each layer.

Melt the butter, mix with the milk, and pour over the potatoes.

Cover the casserole and bake in an oven pre-heated to 350°F/180°C/Gas 4 for 1½ hours. Remove the lid of the casserole and bake for a further 15 minutes.

SNACK PIZZA from 7 months
A quick pizza meal avoiding the preparation of the dough for a base.

---

half a 14 oz (400g) tin of plum tomatoes
2 teaspoons tomato purée
½ teaspoon sweet paprika
1 clove garlic (crushed)
sprig of parsley (chopped)
a little freshly ground black pepper
6 slices wholemeal bread
4 oz (100g) mozzarella cheese
½ a green pepper
1 tomato
8 olives (pitted)

Put the tinned tomatoes, tomato purée, paprika, garlic, parsley and ground pepper into the blender and liquidize.

Chop the green pepper and slice the tomato. Cut the mozzarella into thin strips.

Toast the bread on one side. Turn over the slices, spread the tomato sauce evenly, and top with the cheese pieces, green pepper, tomato and olives. Grill until the cheese starts to melt and brown.

SPANISH BULGHUR from 7 months

---

1 head of sweetcorn (cooked) *or* 4 oz (100g) tinned sweetcorn
1 medium-sized onion
½ a red pepper
½ a green pepper
2 tomatoes
3 dessertspoons olive oil
1 teaspoon sweet paprika
5 oz (150g) bulghur wheat
4 oz (100g) cooked black-eye beans
14 fl oz (400ml) water
1 dessertspoon finely chopped fresh parsley

Scrape the grains of sweetcorn on to a wooden board, using the back of a knife. Peel and dice the onion, wash the peppers and the tomatoes, and chop finely.

Warm the oil in a pan (a heavy-bottomed casserole is best) over a medium heat, and sauté the onion with the paprika for 2–3 minutes until the onion begins to soften.

Add the bulghur and turn with the onion for another 2 minutes. Add the cooked beans and all the vegetables, and pour over the water. Bring to the boil. Cover the pan and simmer over a medium heat for 5 minutes, then reduce the heat and simmer for a further 10 minutes.

Remove from the heat and allow to stand for 5 minutes. Stir in the chopped parsley just before serving.

STUFFED CABBAGE LEAVES

---

4 oz (100g) brown rice and 9 fl oz (250ml) water *or* 6–8 oz
(175–225g) cooked brown rice
½ a small cabbage
2 dessertspoons olive oil
1 large or 2 small carrots
½ a green pepper
6 mushrooms
3 tomatoes
1 medium-sized onion (diced)
1 teaspoon finely chopped fresh oregano
½ teaspoon sweet paprika
2 cloves of garlic (crushed)
1 oz (25g) almonds (ground)
1 oz (25g) grated parmesan cheese

Unless you have sufficient already cooked, cook the rice now
(see page 127).

Meanwhile, wash the cabbage and steam it as a single piece
for 20 minutes. Cool it in a bowl of cold water for a couple of
minutes, then carefully peel apart the larger leaves and drain
(the smaller leaves and the heart can be saved and added to the
stuffing).

Prepare the carrots, pepper, mushrooms and tomatoes,
slicing them all thinly.

Warm the oil and sauté the onion with the oregano, paprika
and garlic for 4–5 minutes until the onion is soft. Add the carrots,
pepper and mushrooms, and stir over a medium heat for a few
minutes. Reduce the heat, add the tomato pieces, cover the pan,
and stew for 5 minutes. Set aside till the rice is cooked.

Pulverize the almonds in a dry blender, and mix with the
parmesan.

Mix the cooked rice and vegetables together, and roll up a
spoonful of the mixture in each of the cabbage leaves.

Arrange the filled leaves in a baking-dish and spoon any
extra stuffing around them.

Sprinkle the almond and parmesan mixture over the top,
and bake in a pre-heated oven at 350°F/180°C/Gas 4 for 20
minutes.

STUFFED POTATOES from 7 months

---

3 large potatoes
6 oz (175g) plain yoghurt
1 teaspoon sweet paprika
3 teaspoons finely chopped fresh chives (or finely diced onion)
1 heaped dessertspoon butter or margarine
2 oz (50g) grated cheddar cheese

Pre-heat the oven to 375°F/190°C/Gas 5.

Scrub the potatoes and score around them with a sharp knife. Bake for 1 hour, then remove from the oven, cut in half along the score, and allow to cool for a few minutes.

Meanwhile, mix the yoghurt, paprika, chives and butter in a bowl. Scoop out the soft centres of the potatoes and add to the mixture. Stir well. Use the mixture to refill the potato skins, top with the cheese, and return to the oven for a further 20 minutes.

SUMMER PEA SOUP

Quick and refreshing, served either hot or cold.

---

a good knob of butter
2 medium-sized onions (diced)
a little freshly ground black pepper
1 dessertspoon each finely chopped fresh chives and thyme
2 good sprigs of fresh mint, finely chopped
10 oz (275g) frozen or shelled fresh peas
10 fl oz (275ml) water
1 dessertspoon lemon juice

Melt the butter over a medium heat, and gently fry the onion till it begins to soften, grinding some pepper over it. Add the herbs, the peas and the water. Bring to the boil and simmer (covered) for 15 minutes.

Add the lemon juice and liquidize.

TOFU CHUNKS from 7 months
The deep-fried chunks of tofu make an excellent finger food, either as a snack or served as a side dish with a main meal of rice and vegetables.

---

8 oz (225g) tofu
2 dessertspoons shoyu
2 dessertspoons water
small piece of fresh ginger root (finely grated)
2 spring onions (finely chopped)
soya oil for deep frying

Cut the tofu into even 1-inch cubes. Mix the shoyu, water, ginger and onions in a bowl for the sauce.

Half fill a pan with oil, and warm over a high to medium heat. The oil must be very hot before the tofu is put in, but should not be allowed to reach smoking-point. Test by dipping one corner of a piece of tofu into the oil: when hot enough, the oil will sizzle on contact. Carefully drop the pieces of tofu into the oil, a few at a time. Stir gently to prevent the chunks sticking together.

When cooked, the tofu will float to the surface of the oil, crisp and just starting to brown. Remove with a perforated spoon and drain on absorbent paper towels.

Serve (to adults) with the previously prepared bowl of sauce as a dip for the chunks of tofu.

VEGETABLE BURGERS from 7 months

It's almost always worth cooking extra quantities of staples such as rice and beans. Here is a recipe using previously cooked rice and beans to make healthy vegetarian burgers to serve on their own or as the filling for a bread roll.

---

1 small onion (finely diced)
2 oz (50g) cabbage (finely chopped)
2 oz (50g) carrots (finely chopped)
1 dessertspoon olive oil
2 dessertspoons shoyu
1 clove garlic (crushed)
6 oz (175g) cooked brown rice
4 oz (100g) cooked kidney beans – other types can be substituted
sprig of fresh parsley (finely chopped)
1 dessertspoon tahini
1 teaspoon brewer's yeast
1 oz (25g) rolled oats (oat flakes)
1 oz (25g) sesame seeds
a little soya oil for frying

Sauté the onion, cabbage and carrot in the olive oil for about 10 minutes until tender. Add the shoyu and garlic and simmer (covered) for a further 5 minutes.

Put the cooked vegetables in a bowl with the rice, beans, parsley, tahini and brewer's yeast, and mix to a paste with your hands. Form into 6 roughly equal balls.

Mix together the oats and the sesame seeds. Roll the balls in the oats and seeds to coat them. Flatten the balls between your hands, and fry gently in soya oil until crisp and browned.

Drain on absorbent paper towels before serving.

VEGETABLE SHEPHERD'S PIE from 7 months

---

6 oz (175g) potatoes
6 oz (175g) carrots
1 dessertspoon olive oil
1 large onion (finely diced)
1 clove garlic (crushed)
a little freshly ground black pepper
4 oz (100g) brown lentils
1 dessertspoon shoyu
8 fl oz (225ml) water
½ a red pepper
2 oz (50g) frozen or shelled fresh peas
2 teaspoons tomato purée
1 dessertspoon tahini

Peel or scrub the potatoes, and scrub the carrots. Boil together till the potatoes are soft.

Meanwhile, warm the oil over a medium heat and fry the onion with the garlic and the ground pepper till lightly browned.

Add the lentils and the shoyu, stir together, and stew (covered) for 2 minutes. Pour over the water, bring to boil, and simmer (covered) over a low heat for 30 minutes.

Stir in the red pepper, the peas, the tomato purée and the tahini. The mixture should be damp but not sloppy. Add a little extra water if necessary. Pour the mixture into a casserole.

Thoroughly mash together the potatoes and the carrots, and put them in a layer over the lentil and vegetable mix. Press down carefully around the edges, and draw a fork across the surface to give a ridged finish.

Bake in a pre-heated oven at 375°F/190°C/Gas 5 for 25–30 minutes.

WHOLEMEAL PIZZA from 7 months

For the base:
1 level teaspoon dried yeast
8 fl oz (225ml) water
11–12 oz (300–350g) wholemeal flour
½ teaspoon salt

For the topping:
half a 14 oz (400g) tin of plum tomatoes
2 teaspoons tomato purée
½ teaspoon sweet paprika
1 clove of garlic (crushed)
sprig of parsley (chopped)
a little freshly ground black pepper
½ a green pepper
1 tomato
4 oz (100g) mozzarella cheese
8 olives (pitted)

Dissolve the yeast in the warm water in a mixing-bowl. Stir in about half the flour, and mix well. Cover the bowl with a cloth and leave to stand in a warm place (an airing-cupboard in winter, a sunny windowsill in summer) for 30–40 minutes.

Stir in the salt and then more flour. Use your hands to knead the dough in the bowl. Form the dough into a rough ball, cover the bowl and leave to stand again for a further 30–40 minutes.

Meanwhile, put the tinned tomatoes, tomato purée, paprika, garlic, parsley and ground pepper into the blender and liquidize.

Chop the green pepper and slice the tomato. Cut the mozzarella into thin strips.

Remove the dough from the bowl and on a flat, floured surface knead it briefly again. It should be soft but not sticky. Work in a little more flour if necessary.

Lightly oil a baking-dish, which should be circular (12 inch diameter), 10 inches square, or equivalent, flat and with a slight lip.

Roll the dough out to a piece a little larger than your

baking-dish. Place it on the dish, trim the edges, and bake in a pre-heated oven at 450°F/230°C/Gas 8 for 5 minutes.

Remove from the oven, spread the tomato sauce evenly over it, and top with the cheese pieces, green pepper, tomato and olives. Return to the oven and bake for a further 20 minutes.

WINTER VEGETABLE STEW from 6 months

---

2 oz (50g) pot barley
10 fl oz (275ml) water
2 oz (50g) brussels sprouts or cabbage
2 oz (50g) carrots (or 1 medium-sized carrot)
2 oz (50g) swede
½ teaspoon miso (fermented soy paste)
½ teaspoon brewer's yeast

Wash the barley and put it in a pan with the water. Bring to the boil, then reduce the heat and simmer (covered) for about 30 minutes, when the grains will be soft through. (Polished or 'pearl' barley is a more refined product, and has a shorter cooking time – about 20 minutes.)

Meanwhile, prepare the vegetables. Sprouts can be used whole, but wash them thoroughly and cut away any discoloured or damaged outer leaves. Wash and roughly chop cabbage. Scrub or peel the carrots and peel the swede. Roughly dice the root vegetables.

Add all the vegetables to the cooked barley and simmer (covered) for a further 10–12 minutes. The vegetables should still be firm, but soft enough to cut with a table-knife.

For a child up to about 8 months, or until he is happy with finger foods, remove what he will eat at this stage and blend it, adding a little soya milk if necessary to achieve a smooth consistency.

Add the miso just before serving, making sure that it dissolves and is evenly distributed.

Index

FOR THE BEST IN PAPERBACKS, LOOK FOR THE

In every corner of the world, on every subject under the sun, Penguin represents quality and variety – the very best in publishing today.

For complete information about books available from Penguin – including Puffins, Penguin Classics and Arkana – and how to order them, write to us at the appropriate address below. Please note that for copyright reasons the selection of books varies from country to country.

In the United Kingdom: Please write to *Dept E.P., Penguin Books Ltd, Harmondsworth, Middlesex, UB7 0DA.*

If you have any difficulty in obtaining a title, please send your order with the correct money, plus ten per cent for postage and packaging, to *PO Box No 11, West Drayton, Middlesex*

In the United States: Please write to *Dept BA, Penguin, 299 Murray Hill Parkway, East Rutherford, New Jersey 07073*

In Canada: Please write to *Penguin Books Canada Ltd, 2801 John Street, Markham, Ontario L3R 1B4*

In Australia: Please write to the *Marketing Department, Penguin Books Australia Ltd, P.O. Box 257, Ringwood, Victoria 3134*

In New Zealand: Please write to the *Marketing Department, Penguin Books (NZ) Ltd, Private Bag, Takapuna, Auckland 9*

In India: Please write to *Penguin Overseas Ltd, 706 Eros Apartments, 56 Nehru Place, New Delhi, 110019*

In the Netherlands: Please write to *Penguin Books Nederland B.V., Postbus 195, NL–1380AD Weesp*

In West Germany: Please write to *Penguin Books Ltd, Friedrichstrasse 10–12, D–6000 Frankfurt/Main 1*

In Spain: Please write to *Longman Penguin España, Calle San Nicolas 15, E–28013 Madrid*

In Italy: Please write to *Penguin Italia s.r.l., Via Como 4, I-20096 Pioltello (Milano)*

In France: Please write to *Penguin Books Ltd, 39 Rue de Montmorency, F-75003 Paris*

In Japan: Please write to *Longman Penguin Japan Co Ltd, Yamaguchi Building, 2–12–9 Kanda Jimbocho, Chiyoda-Ku, Tokyo 101*

PENGUIN HEALTH

Audrey Eyton's F-Plus   Audrey Eyton

'Your short cut to the most sensational diet of the century' – *Daily Express*

Baby and Child   Penelope Leach

A beautifully illustrated and comprehensive handbook on the first five years of life. 'It stands head and shoulders above anything else available at the moment' – Mary Kenny in the *Spectator*

Woman's Experience of Sex   Sheila Kitzinger

Fully illustrated with photographs and line drawings, this book explores the riches of women's sexuality at every stage of life. 'A book which any mother could confidently pass on to her daughter – and her partner too' – *Sunday Times*

Food Additives   Erik Millstone

Eat, drink and be worried? Erik Millstone's hard-hitting book contains powerful evidence about the massive risks being taken with the health of the consumer. It takes the lid off food and the food industry.

Living with Allergies   Dr John McKenzie

At least 20% of the population suffer from an allergic disorder at some point in their lives and this invaluable book provides accurate and up-to-date information about the condition, where to go for help, diagnosis and cure – and what we can do to help ourselves.

Living with Stress   Cary L. Cooper, Rachel D. Cooper and Lynn H. Eaker

Stress leads to more stress, and the authors of this helpful book show why low levels of stress are desirable and how best we can achieve them in today's world. Looking at those most vulnerable, they demonstrate ways of breaking the vicious circle that can ruin lives.

PENGUIN HEALTH

Living with Asthma and Hay Fever   John Donaldson

For the first time, there are now medicines that can prevent asthma attacks from taking place. Based on up-to-date research, this book shows how the majority of sufferers can beat asthma and hay fever and lead full and active lives.

Anorexia Nervosa   R. L. Palmer

Lucid and sympathetic guidance for those who suffer from this disturbing illness, and for their families and professional helpers, given with a clarity and compassion that will make anorexia more understandable and consequently less frightening for everyone involved.

Medicines: A Guide for Everybody   Peter Parish

This sixth edition of a comprehensive survey of all the medicines available over the counter or on prescription offers clear guidance for the ordinary reader as well as invaluable information for those involved in health care.

Pregnancy and Childbirth   Sheila Kitzinger

A complete and up-to-date guide to physical and emotional preparation for pregnancy – a must for all prospective parents.

The Penguin Encyclopaedia of Nutrition   John Yudkin

This book cuts through all the myths about food and diets to present the real facts clearly and simply. 'Everyone should buy one' – *Nutrition News and Notes*

The Parents' A to Z   Penelope Leach

For anyone with children of 6 months, 6 years or 16 years, this guide to all the little problems involved in their health, growth and happiness will prove reassuring and helpful.

PENGUIN HEALTH

Positive Smear Susan Quilliam

A 'positive' cervical smear result is not only a medical event but an emotional event too: one which means facing up to issues surrounding your sexuality, fertility and mortality. Based on personal experiences, Susan Quilliam's practical guide will help every woman meet that challenge.

Medicine The Self-Help Guide
Professor Michael Orme and Dr Susanna Grahame-Jones

A new kind of home doctor – with an entirely new approach. With a unique emphasis on self-management, *Medicine* takes an *active* approach to drugs, showing how to maximize their benefits, speed up recovery and minimize dosages through self-help and non-drug alternatives.

Defeating Depression Tony Lake

Counselling, medication and the support of friends can all provide invaluable help in relieving depression. But if we are to combat it once and for all we must face up to perhaps painful truths about our past and take the first steps forward that can eventually transform our lives. This lucid and sensitive book shows us how.

Freedom and Choice in Childbirth Sheila Kitzinger

Undogmatic, honest and compassionate, Sheila Kitzinger's book raises searching questions about the kind of care offered to the pregnant woman – and will help her make decisions and communicate effectively about the kind of birth experience she desires.

Care of the Dying Richard Lamerton

It is never true that 'nothing more can be done' for the dying. This book shows us how to face death without pain, with humanity, with dignity and in peace.

PENGUIN HEALTH

Healing Nutrients   Patrick Quillin

A guide to using the vitamins and minerals contained in everyday foods to fight off disease and promote well-being: to prevent common ailments, cure some of the more destructive diseases, reduce the intensity of others, augment conventional treatment and speed up healing.

Total Relaxation in Five Steps   Louis Proto

With Louis Proto's Alpha Plan you can counteract stress, completely relaxing both mind and body, in just 30 minutes a day. By reaching the Alpha state – letting the feelings, senses and imagination predominate – even the most harassed can feel totally rejuvenated.

Aromatherapy for Everyone   Robert Tisserand

The use of aromatic oils in massage can relieve many ailments and alleviate stress and related symptoms.

Spiritual and Lay Healing   Philippa Pullar

An invaluable new survey of the history of healing that sets out to separate the myths from the realities.

Hypnotherapy for Everyone   Dr Ruth Lever

This book demonstrates that hypnotherapy is a real alternative to conventional healing methods in many ailments.

FOR THE BEST IN PAPERBACKS, LOOK FOR THE 🐧

FROM THE PENGUIN COOKERY LIBRARY

The Best of Eliza Acton   Selected and Edited by Elizabeth Ray
With an Introduction by Elizabeth David

First published in 1845, Eliza Acton's *Modern Cookery for Private Families*, of which this is a selection, is a true classic which everyone interested in cookery will treasure.

Easy to Entertain   Patricia Lousada

Easy to Entertain hands you the magic key to entertaining without days of panic or last minute butterflies. The magic lies in cooking each course ahead, so that you can enjoy yourself along with your guests.

French Provincial Cooking   Elizabeth David

'It is difficult to think of any home that can do without Elizabeth David's *French Provincial Cooking* ... One could cook for a lifetime on the book alone' – *Observer*

The National Trust Book of Traditional Puddings   Sara Paston-Williams

'My favourite cookbook of the year. Engagingly written ... this manages to be both scholarly and practical, elegant without pretension' – *Sunday Times*

The New Book of Middle Eastern Food   Claudia Roden

'This is one of those rare cookery books that is a work of cultural anthropology and Mrs Roden's standards of scholarship are so high as to ensure that it has permanent value' – Paul Levy in the *Observer*

Charcuterie and French Pork Cookery   Jane Grigson

'Fully comprehensive ... a detailed and enlightening insight into the preparation and cooking of pork. Altogether a unique book' – *Wine and Food*. 'The research is detailed, the recounting lively, the information fascinating' – *The Times*

FOR THE BEST IN PAPERBACKS, LOOK FOR THE

FROM THE PENGUIN COOKERY LIBRARY

North Atlantic Seafood   Alan Davidson

'A classic work of reference and a cook's delight' (*The Times Educational Supplement*) from the world's greatest expert on fish cookery. 'Mr Davidson has a gift for conveying memorable information in a way so effortless that his book makes lively reading for its own sake' – Elizabeth David

The Foods and Wines of Spain   Penelope Casas

'I have not come across a book before that captures so well the unlikely medieval mix of Eastern and Northern, earthy and fine, rare and deeply familiar ingredients that make up the Spanish kitchen' – *Harpers and Queen*. 'The definitive book on Spanish cooking ... a jewel in the crown of culinary literature' – Craig Claiborne

An Omelette and a Glass of Wine   Elizabeth David

'She has the intelligence, subtlety, sensuality, courage and creative force of the true artist' – *Wine and Food*. 'Her pieces are so entertaining, so original, often witty, critical yet lavish with their praise, that they succeed in enthusing even the most jaded palate' – Arabella Boxer in *Vogue*

English Food   Jane Grigson

'Jane Grigson is perhaps the most serious and discriminating of her generation of cookery writers, and *English Food* is an anthology all who follow her recipes will want to buy for themselves as well as for friends who may wish to know about *real* English food ... enticing from page to page' – Pamela Vandyke Price in the *Spectator*

Classic Cheese Cookery   Peter Graham

Delicious, mouth-watering soups, starters, main meals and desserts using cheeses from throughout Europe make this tempting cookery book a must for everyone with an interest in the subject. Clear, informative and comprehensive, it is a book to return to again and again.